WHAT PEOPLE ARE

THE CASE OF THE DISA

In this fascinating symposium of case history and personal experience Dr Heyse-Moore has underlined the two-way bridge between patient and physician. It is an important addition to the library of hospice medicine and palliative care.

But there is more: meditate on each story separately and you may find memories of your own recalled... and brought to life.
Dr Tom West OBE, former Medical Director St Christopher's Hospice.

With the skill of the age-old storyteller Louis takes us on a perambulation, a 'walkabout' through the songlines of his encounters and chance meetings.

Using what he refers to as the 'feel-see' quality of the Hawaiian shaman, Louis' layering of his painterly observations and the slow ease of his storytelling style drop us into a space where we hover between time past and time present.

He knits together the broken body with the soulful healing that comes from being seen, heard, and recognised body-to-body. These seemingly simple stories work to promote 'wholeness' and a sense of well-being in his readers. Louis' mythopoetic style envelops us in the very healing process that he is describing.
Marian Dunlea, Jungian analyst, Somatic Experiencing trauma therapist, faculty member Marion Woodman Foundation.

The Case of the Disappearing Cancer

And other stories of illness and healing, life and death

The Case of the Disappearing Cancer

And other stories of illness
and healing, life and death

Louis Heyse-Moore

AYNI
BOOKS

Winchester, UK
Washington, USA

First published by Ayni Books, 2014
Ayni Books is an imprint of John Hunt Publishing Ltd., Laurel House, Station Approach,
Alresford, Hants, SO24 9JH, UK
office1@jhpbooks.net
www.johnhuntpublishing.com
www.ayni-books.com

For distributor details and how to order please visit the 'Ordering' section on our website.

Text copyright: Louis Heyse-Moore 2013

ISBN: 978 1 78279 614 5

All rights reserved. Except for brief quotations in critical articles or reviews, no part of this
book may be reproduced in any manner without prior written permission from the publishers.

The rights of Louis Heyse-Moore as author have been asserted in accordance with the Copyright,
Designs and Patents Act 1988.

A CIP catalogue record for this book is available from the British Library.

Design: Stuart Davies

Printed and bound by CPI Group (UK) Ltd, Croydon, CR0 4YY

We operate a distinctive and ethical publishing philosophy in all
areas of our business, from our global network of authors to
production and worldwide distribution.

CONTENTS

Dedication
To Joan
and to Matthew, Dominique and Gabrielle

By the same author

Speaking of Dying: A Practical Guide to Using Counselling Skills in Palliative Care

Hope is the thing with feathers
That perches in the soul...
Emily Dickinson (1924) from poem XXXII

Tell me, O Muse, of the man of many devices, who wandered
full many ways... aye, and many the woes he suffered in his
heart upon the sea, seeking to win his own life and the return
of his comrades.
Homer, The Odyssey (1919, p. 3)

Acknowledgements

My thanks to my wife Joan, whose down-to-earth critiques have been invaluable, who bore patiently with the many hours I spent writing and rewriting this book and who has been my companion on our journeys of exploration. My thanks, too, to my sister, Joanna, for reading the manuscript and for her supportive comments; and to my sister Damaris whose story I told with her permission in "The Inner Tyre".

Introduction

I am on a healing journey, driving with my wife, Joan, through a forest in Fiji. It is late and the light is fading. Tall, dark trees line the dirt track; all around us is silent woodland with occasional open spaces for crops. Our car sways as we drive over potholes and its tyres crunch on stones. It is the rainy season. The air is close and humid, and carries the smell of damp earth from recent torrential rain. We are looking for a tiny village somewhere in this enchanted forest.

It began, I suppose, about twenty years ago when my father died suddenly. I still remember my wife's phone call to tell me of his death. I can recall how I felt: the mixture of shock, grief and a kind of inner shaking as if some earthquake were rumbling inside me. And I can still see the pale, washed-blue morning sky which I stared at outside my office window as she spoke.

Years later I find myself going through boxes of old family photographs and documents. They include many of my father's early life – he was born in 1912 on a plantation in Fiji – and I look with fascination at the old sepia images of a past age. In one he is perhaps six months old, and is being held by his Indian ayah while his older brother looks on; they sit on a rug made of some animal skin. In another, the family are having a picnic by the sea. The beach is deserted and the forest comes down close to the sand. The women are in Edwardian dresses, the men in whites with boaters or straw hats. Other pictures show him in front of the plantation house built on stilts that he and his family lived in. There are pictures of teams of buffaloes, guided by Indian plantation workers, pulling carts loaded with sugar cane, and of large rafts, steered by Fijians, piled high with sugar cane, drifting down the river to the sugar mills.

My father, although he talked of returning to Fiji and Australia where he grew up, never did make the journey. So we, his children, only knew him as an emigrant from his place of birth.

A year further on, after months of research, I am in a plane flying six miles above the Pacific Ocean at night. Joan sleeps beside me. Wakeful, I look out of the window and see the vast bowl of the black night sky stippled with stars, the moon's silver reflection on the wing of the plane and long cloud ribs set out like herringbones below us. I shiver. It has the feel of magic. I am completing an incomplete circle on behalf of my father and myself.

A few days later, we are sitting on rattan matting on the floor in a village hall – we have found the village. Everyone there has turned out to greet us. Our gifts have been accepted. The headman makes a speech in Fijian and local chiefs follow. We drink kava[1] from a huge stone ceremonial bowl. I tell my story. They sing. I show my old photographs. The oldest man there is in tears – he can just remember the bullock carts used to transport the sugar cane nearly eighty years ago. They are not at all surprised that I have journeyed to my father's birthplace. Ancestry is very important to them. It is only right to honour one's father in this way. The old plantation house, though, is long gone – destroyed by termites – but it doesn't matter. The circle has been completed.

Healing is the theme of this book, and how it can be found in the most unlikely places. I have always loved stories about people who painstakingly reconstruct a ruined building or who, with infinite care, clean away the dirt and overpainting from some old, faded, grimy painting to reveal a thing of beauty underneath. Healing is something like this. Just as a physical wound knits together, so our scattered and divided memories and feelings and experiences can knit together to form a pattern, a wholeness encompassing both light and shade.

Once, on a sweltering afternoon, I visited the city of Ravenna in Italy. I stepped into the cool, quiet darkness of one of the 6th century AD churches and was astonished by the beautiful, luminous mosaics. In one, white doves perched on the edge of a bowl of water, while in another egrets hunted in rivers. In yet another, golden stars lit up the dark blue heavens. Saints and angels, Christ and his mother Mary, and the three Magi were revealed in splendour adorning the walls and ceilings and cupolas. Everywhere were geometric patterns and repeating leafy shapes. And all of this was created from millions of tiny pieces of differently coloured stone chips – antique pixels of light and shade.

Healing is not a passive process. Of course minor cuts and grazes heal seemingly of their own accord. Healing from a major illness, however, needs our participation. It is something we engage in actively. It can be hard work. And it is about all of us, body, mind, soul and relationships. Furthermore, it isn't something we can just pay lip service to; whole-heartedness is a must. Proust (2006, p. 131) wrote: "Illness is the doctor to whom we pay most heed; to kindness, to knowledge, we make promises only; pain we obey.

And if we don't, we're in trouble.

Stories are the substance of this book. Many of them are about people I have known as a doctor, who have experienced significant illness, and either got better, lived with chronic sickness or went on to die. In all of them the search for meaning was present in some fashion, even if it was not explicated. It made its presence felt as one might feel the vibration underfoot of an underground tube train while walking along a London pavement. It might present itself in any guise – religious, spiritual, philosophical or secular. And it was as insistent as waves rolling up a beach.

And I was in some way a part of their story, discovering meaning with them and connecting with them, whether as listener, witness, doctor, counsellor or narrator. "No man is an island, entire of itself," said John Donne (1839, pp. 574–5). In Buddhism there is a beautiful image which describes our connectedness. In the heavenly home of the Vedic God, Indra, there is a multidimensional net of infinite size, which may be seen as a metaphor for the whole Universe. At each knot, a shining jewel is hung; reflected in each mirror-like jewel are all the other jewels in the net, infinite in number. Furthermore, each of the jewels reflected in this way itself reflects all the other jewels. Everything and everyone is connected. Healing is for the bits that aren't.

I have always lived in a medical ambience. Since my father was a surgeon, we – that is me, my brother and my two sisters – grew up in the 1950s with the realities of life with a doctor. In addition to his hospital work, he had private patients who came to our house, so we had to keep out of their way – and keep quiet too. His consulting room (which we nicknamed his sulking room) smelt of antiseptic and contained the mysterious paraphernalia of his work – steel surgical instruments, sterilising equipment, hypodermic syringes, an examination couch and so on. His office was decidedly a medical room, stamped with his personality. He would sit at his desk writing up his notes (such terrible handwriting) and smoking a cigar. Even today I have only to smell the smoke of a Havana and in a moment I am back there again.

It's not surprising, then, that I went into medicine. But there was more to my choosing than I realised at the time. Healing, despite another strong contender, must be humanity's oldest calling. From the time we became human, wherever a group of people lived together there was a constant need for healing – of hunting wounds, infections, broken bones, possession by evil spirits and so on. Those with an aptitude would be singled out to develop their skills further: hence the shamans and medicine persons of traditional cultures. Further, they would choose an apprentice to learn their skills and continue their tradition after they had died. This is a familiar pattern in many traditional societies.

When I read the Hippocratic Oath, I find myself touched by the part that describes this:

> I will pay the same respect to my master in the Science as to my parents and share my life with him… I will regard his sons as my brothers and teach them the Science, if they desire to learn it… I will hand on precepts, lectures and all other learning to my sons, to those of my master and to those pupils duly apprenticed and sworn…
> (Porter 1997, p. 63)

This played out, I think, between my father and me. When I became a medical student, he and I would have lengthy medical discussions. I attended his ward rounds sometimes and watched him operating. I even attended a post mortem with him. And when I was struggling to understand some point of anatomy before an exam (there were a lot of those), he would patiently explain it to me.

As a newly qualified doctor I first saw the body as an object to be observed, examined, tested and treated. Now, as a counsellor working with traumatised people, I still focus on the body, but in a different way. As I sit with a client, we become aware, yet again, of the animal nature of our bodies and how they speak to us if only we know how to listen. The brittle smile, the spontaneous belly laugh, the lump in the throat, the heaviness in the chest, hands placed protectively in front of the stomach, chills running down the spine. The messages are there to be read if we attend. Stroll along a crowded street and watch the way people walk, how they hold their bodies, what they do with their arms and the expressions on their faces – sad, angry, blank, laughing, frozen, curious, bored – it's like a book. We can't help communicating.

A few years after I qualified, I went to a conference at St Christopher's Hospice on symptom control. This was back in the 1970s when the modern hospice movement was still in its infancy and St Christopher's was just becoming known as a centre of excellence in terminal care, as it was then known. I remember two speakers particularly. One was Dr Mary Baines, one of the consultants there. She spoke with clarity and authority about the practicalities of successful relief of pain and other symptoms such as breathlessness and vomiting. Her talk was like a recipe book, precise, tried and tested, and effective. Nothing quite like this had been around before. Looking after dying people in hospital had sometimes felt to me like a nightmare; the symptom control hit or miss. Here at last was an approach that worked. I felt a huge sense of relief. Then Dr Tom West, the Deputy Medical Director, spoke about the patients in the hospice. He did so in a way completely different from the usual medical lecture. He told us stories – stories about their illnesses, stories to illustrate the different kinds of pain, stories about the effects of good symptom control on the lives of patients. His was an unashamedly personal approach and the individual patients sprang vividly to life as he spoke.

The day was an awakening for me. It opened my mind to a new way of thinking. Like so many advances it seemed obvious in hindsight. Their approach was practical and compassionate. Suffering, both physical and psychological, was seen as something significant and important, not to be just tolerated but to be addressed and alleviated as a worthy end in itself. Within a year I went into hospice medicine.

I soon discovered, however, that this was no easy option. I was, after all, working with the dying. However, I also found that people close to death may become intensely alive. Only the essentials remain, the rest falls away. Time spent with family and friends became infinitely precious. Late nights at the office became a distant, even irrelevant, memory.

I became aware of a paradox: you can be healed yet not cured, and, conversely, cured yet not healed. There are healthy ways of being ill and there are healthy ways of dying – and there are even unhealthy ways of being cured, like alcoholics who have had a liver transplant and go back to drinking.

Cure is often conceptualised in terms of fighting a war. Deadly cancers are excised, blocked arteries are reamed out, abscesses are incised, collections of blood compressing the brain are drained, broken bones are set, hearts are transplanted. Antibiotics – first known as magic bullets – destroy invading armies of bacteria, antidepressants brighten our sagging neurones, insulin props up the failing pancreas, chemothera-peutic agents surge through the body destroying malignant cells by the billion and are supported by bombardments of radio-therapy.

Healing, however, is different. It comes from the Old English *haelen*, meaning whole or well. If curing is about destroying the enemy, healing is about putting back together the fragmented chaos that reigns after the battle. But we need also to go beyond the physical. Minds get traumatised, families split, souls go through dark nights and our environment is raped. They all require their own healing. All these elements are interrelated, a five-sided cat's cradle: pull on one thread and all the others will be affected, whether for good or ill.

As a medical student, I used to imagine the physician as a powerful technician of the body, a skilled, invulnerable warrior combating ferocious diseases. The thing was, I didn't feel like that at all. As a newly qualified doctor I felt inexperienced and vulnerable. I certainly didn't feel powerful – I kept making mistakes and having to swallow my pride and ask for help. Many patients' illnesses responded to treatment just as set out in the textbooks but, sadly, many didn't. I was faced with the limits of medicine.

It was a character from Greek mythology that taught me a lesson about this. Chiron the centaur was a great healer He had been incurably wounded in his leg by a deadly poisoned arrow, yet being immortal he could not die. His long search for a cure increased his skills as a healer manifold. And the sick flocked to him; they knew he understood their suffering.

We (and that includes doctors) have all had some illness, some trauma, some loss, some tragedy in our lives. This should not be a matter of shame. What we have experienced, or maybe still experience, helps us to recognise what our patient or client or friend is going through. Our vulnerability, then, becomes our strength and our point of connection with the sick.

Healing in its wider sense is not the exclusive preserve of doctors. It is a gift we are all born with; it's just that we often don't recognise it. It may happen in the simplest ways, so ordinary that it is not even noticed. And yet it is everywhere. Perhaps Buddhists have a contribution here: they speak of mindfulness, a constant awareness of all we do, where each happening is noted and valued and released, and where the sacredness of life is recognised in even the smallest occurrences. Then pouring a cup of tea, listening to a friend or visiting someone who is sick all become healing moments.

This book is for anyone who has ever experienced illness or loss, whether in person or indirectly through a relative or friend. It is for anyone who has experienced any of the traumas that life may bring, whether small or large. It is for people who are on a journey of healing. It is, too, for the professionals who work with ill or dying people and who listen to their extraordinary stories day in and day out.

Identifying details of patient and client examples have been changed to preserve anonymity. The only exception is the story of

Bill Ellis in "The Eagle and the Mountain", because he 'went public' with his autobiography.

Chapter 1

The Case of the Disappearing Cancer

The referral seemed quite straightforward: a request for home support for a woman with advanced, metastatic cancer. I noted from information given that she had a huge tumour filling perhaps a third of her abdomen along with widespread secondary tumours. From previous experience with patients with a similar story, I thought she would be very ill and might need admission to the hospice soon. I rang the doorbell of her maisonette. A slim, fit-looking woman in her early fifties answered the door. I explained who I was and asked if I might see the patient. "Oh, that's me," she said. I was nonplussed – I had expected someone much sicker. However, we sat down and went through the history of her illness and the hospital investigations she had had, including a biopsy which proved the diagnosis. It was when I examined her that I began to think something strange was going on. Where there had been a massive tumour, there was now almost nothing to feel.

I explained to her what I had found – or rather not found. I was in the strange position of telling someone who had been informed she was dying that this was not the case. I had to choose my words carefully. I didn't want to build her hopes up too much before further tests had clarified what was happening. I ended by saying, rather obviously, that she didn't need palliative care and that I would speak to her general practitioner. She remained very calm throughout our meeting, almost as though she knew what I would say. When I spoke to her general practitioner later that day, I suggested rerunning her tests. He referred her back to hospital and the further investigations showed that her metastases had disappeared and that her abdominal tumour had shrunk right down. They followed her with serial scans which showed a continuing reduction in the size of the mass. Eventually they did a further biopsy which showed only scar tissue.

I went back to see her to talk over these results. She didn't have any explanation for what had happened. In fact, she was politely reluctant to talk about it. I knew that her spirituality was very important to her and I wondered if she had experienced something that she preferred to keep private. She did say, however, that one day during her illness she knew she was going to be all right. A year later I went back to see her. She remained well and, when I examined her, there was no sign of any recurrence. Her hospital medical team wrote her case up in a medical journal as an example of spontaneous regression of cancer.

Such a story, I thought to myself after seeing her. Cancer just doesn't do that. But, in this case, it did. I found myself shaking my head and smiling. I felt awed. I was reminded of those lines from *Hamlet*: "There are more things in Heaven and Earth, Horatio, than are dreamt of in your philosophy." (Shakespeare: *Hamlet*. 1:5:166–7) Calling it a spontaneous remission didn't help much. All that meant in plain English was that she had got better of her own accord, which we knew already; it wasn't a diagnosis.

When I talked to other doctors about it, they would listen politely and then change the subject. This always surprised me. If a patient had been given a drug which had caused an advanced cancer to shrink away permanently with no side effects over a matter of weeks and with no recurrence on follow-up, it would have been headline news around the world, equivalent, perhaps, to the discovery of penicillin. So, why was there so little interest here? There are, after all, many other similar cases reported in the medical literature. Surely they are important.

The thing is, these reports don't fit with our present clinical understanding of how advanced cancer behaves. We imagine it as inexorable, malign, like a host of black crabs that keep coming back. Yet, in rare cases, it just melts away. So here is a phenomenon that in medical terms has not been explained, cannot be predicted and cannot be controlled. It is well documented clinically and yet has the feel of being on the fringe of medicine. Perhaps it is not so surprising that doctors are cautious of exploring it.

I see such stories as signposts. Understanding the mechanism of such occasional spontaneous remissions is still speculative[2] and, of course, many people continue to die from advanced cancer. But these strange cancer regressions have a message for the future. Maybe there will be a way of healing cancer which will not involve the often gruelling surgery, chemotherapy and radiotherapy necessary at the moment, an approach that may be as radically different as antibiotics are from the old practice of bloodletting for the treatment of infections.

What must it be like, though, to find you aren't dying after all? Perhaps it would be like coming up for air, as if from a deep dive underwater. Or climbing out of a dank cave with its sharp, cold stone smells into blue sky, sunlight, and soft air. A sense of elation, freedom, of being able to breathe, of lightness, of being alive. Or perhaps it might feel overwhelming at first, even disorientating; perhaps you'd be in a state of shock for days or weeks and only gradually would the sweetness of what has happened filter in. Perhaps you'd feel sorrow because you've recovered and so many haven't. You'd realise that you will not be taken from your spouse or your children and then, why, you could not get enough of being with them; they are so precious to you. Suddenly you have to think of living again, being able to go out shopping, go for a walk, go on holiday; get a job even. Perhaps you'd be so elated you'd want to tell the world about it; or maybe you'd prefer to stay quiet, say as little as possible for fear of being thought a freak. Perhaps you'd want to do something – work for a cancer charity, set one up, go skydiving or write a book to raise funds, whatever moves you – as a sign of your gratitude. Perhaps your whole view of life would be altered.

Such remarkable healings are rare. More often, healing comes in more subtle ways: over days or years; in part or in whole; or remitting, healing and illness alternating in a slow dance. It may be not only of our body but also of our mind, our relationships or our soul. Or maybe our body continues in its illness while our psyche is transformed. What follows are stories about the multi-faceted and surprising nature of healing.

Chapter 2

Discovering Life

When my children were young they used to play with sticks of Plasticine of different colours. Sometimes I joined in and I remember the particular smell of the Plasticine, the satisfying perfect smoothness of the new pieces, which were either tube-shaped or like short corrugated rulers. I recall, too, the way all the colours started to mix up together after the pieces had been used a few times, and the look of intense concentration on my children's faces as they worked at their creations. One of the figures that children often make is of a person, a simple human figure with head, body and limbs. They might take this inanimate model and bring it to life, make it walk, moving the legs with their hands. Or they might make the arms move to carry out some task. And they would provide a voice as this little Plasticine figure met and talked to other toys.

The story of the creation of the first humans in Genesis has surprising similarities. God takes some clay and makes Adam, the first man. Then he breathes on his creation, and, lo and behold, Adam comes to life. He takes a rib from Adam's side while Adam is asleep (the first anaesthetic; lucky fellow) and makes Eve. Job done.

This seems at first glance a childlike story and yet, even today, in our scientific age there is no unequivocal delineation of what exactly life is. In scientific terms we may talk about characteristics of life such as homeostasis, growth and reproduction. These, however, are descriptions, not explanations. While life is something so familiar that we take it for granted, it is, nevertheless, mysterious. We talk about feeling alive, or, alternatively, feeling like death warmed up. If we find we have a life-threatening illness we fight for our life; it is sweet to us and we want it to continue.

I remember one experience I had that taught me that life is more than just a series of biochemical reactions. Joan and I were on holiday on Kauai, one of the Hawaiian Islands. We decided to visit Polihale, a remote beach on the west of the island. To get there we had a five-mile hike along a dirt track. On our left were huge dunes, some a hundred feet high covered with bushes and trees. On our right was a wide tongue of flat land that used to be a swamp and was now given over to crops. Clouds of twittering songbirds rose and fell among the corn. Mountains rose behind in stepped ranks leading to the volcanic crater over 5000 feet above us at the centre of the island. Then a Hawaiian drove past and offered us a lift in his gleaming black 4WD. A quarter of an hour later we walked out on to the north end of the beach.

It was overwhelming. My first impression was of huge space. The beach was enormous, 100 yards wide, and I knew it stretched for 17 miles southwards. The breakers from the sea roared as they swept up the sand. This blended with the sound of the wind blowing cooling, salty air from the sea. I looked up at the cliffs to the north. We felt dwarfed by their vast presence rising hundreds of feet above us. Their dark grey blunt volcanic stone headlands, horizontally ribbed, marched away in serried ranks from where the beach ended. We stood there and looked with awe at this massive, natural spectacle.

I remember breathing in the clean, fresh, saline air and feeling my whole body – not just my lungs – expand and soften, as though an ancient constriction had been shed like a redundant skin. I felt – there is no other word for it – alive. The sky was blue with a few clouds sailing by bringing alternating sun and shade. I looked along the miles of sand. We had the beach to ourselves. It was so beautiful I found it hard to believe there were no tourists. We took our walking shoes off and tied them to our rucksacks. I still remember how my bare feet slid luxuriously into the soft, granular, coral sand. Ahead of us we could see multiple tyre tracks leading away along the beach. I wondered if these were made by local Hawaiians racing their 4WDs at night.

We walked slowly along the beach, our paired footprints veering down towards the wet golden sand, where they sank deep, and then to the surf from the waves, which washed them away as if they had never been. We could have been the first, or only, man and woman on the planet. It was altogether pleasurable.

I looked back after a while and could just see the 4WD in the distance and people standing beside it. They looked tiny, black dots on the pale yellow sand at the base of the huge cliffs above them. Like nothing else this gave me a sense of the immense scale of the place.

Of course, our bodies were biochemically alive and functioned in their usual way. But this experience was more than that. I could actually taste life like a fruit. When I breathed, I wasn't just taking in oxygen, I felt as if I were inhaling life itself. I had, for a little, woken up and become aware of a miracle.

To me, then, when the writers of Genesis spoke of the breath of God animating Adam's clay body, they were referring to a profound mystery. I can think of dying people I have known who overflowed with life and, by contrast, other people who were physically well but seemed to be half-dead, grey, frozen and withdrawn. Life, as I see it, is more than just our physiology; it imbues and gives meaning to every aspect of our existence, body, feelings, mind and soul.

The Breath of Life

Spirit is, among other things, an air word.

Every time I attended the labour ward, life was writ large over the drama being played out. The room was always kept at a tropical heat so that the newly born babies wouldn't become hypothermic. The mother-to-be would be lying on the delivery bed in some disarray, her hospital gown and sterile drapes rucked over her abdomen, her knees drawn up and, all modesty lost, her genitalia exposed to the powerful light trained on them. Every minute or two another contraction would come on. She would be sweating and groaning with the pain and the effort of pushing down, encouraged by her husband and one of the nurses, who would be holding her arms to give her purchase as she strained. At the end of labour, the baby's head appeared and in a moment he slithered out between his mother's legs covered in body fluids and soft white vernix. There was a tense pause. Would he breathe? His exhausted mother would be watching anxiously as the midwife sucked mucus from her baby's mouth and nostrils with a tube. Then there came a spluttering cry and I could feel the apprehension in the room evaporate. He was all right. The moment when her new baby was returned to the mother was always very moving. She would be smiling, and sometimes crying at the same time. The tenderness with which she held her child was palpable. Her husband, beside her, would be staring at his new son, wide-eyed and speechless. Sometimes he would be in tears too. I never grew tired of this scene no matter how often I watched it or how fatigued I was.

Just occasionally the baby was not all right and, limp, pale and not breathing, she would be brought over to me, the on-call paediatrician, to resuscitate her. I would go into emergency mode as I worked on her, providing artificial ventilation to oxygenate her lungs. After the initial crisis, I would watch fascinated and entranced as her skin changed from pale grey to pink, as she started to move her limbs and she began to breathe and cry – it was as though she was coming to life before my eyes. And best of all was to see her returned to her mother. I was always aware, as I resuscitated her child, of her eyes watching, frightened, sometimes tearful, sometimes frozen. I would watch happily as her baby was returned to her and see her changing expressions – mingled relief and joy – as she held her daughter safely in her arms for the first time.

If we look for the first breath in of a newborn, we look with equal intensity for the last breath out of the dying. Whenever I have been with someone close to death, I've been aware how the family, perhaps not knowing what else to expect, carefully watched the dying person's breathing. For them, this was the moment of death.

While it is obvious we need oxygen to survive, there is, I think, something more going on here. The word spirit comes for the Latin *spiritus*, meaning breath and also soul, courage and vigour. (Chambers 1988) In other words, the source of life was considered to be the air. It wasn't just a gas, it was life itself. How did this idea come about?

In 1994, two cave explorers in Chauvet in Southern France were investigating a small passageway blocked with debris on the side of a gorge and stumbled on a hidden complex of caves. They discovered a wealth of extraordinary cave paintings, up to 35,000 years old. (Clottes 2003) These included maneless lions which roamed that region then, along with pictures of the animals they hunted – horses, deer, and the huge, aggressive aurochs. The artists would have watched these predators pursuing and throttling their prey. They knew very well that breathing and life were intimately connected. It would have been but a short step to deduce that the air they breathed was also the source of their vitality. Our present day language still contains echoes of this. Inspiration can mean breathing in but it can also mean to be inspired. Expiration means to breathe out, but it also means to die. It's telling that when a person has a cardiac arrest, we still talk of giving her the kiss of life. The life-giving oxygen in our lungs is transferred in this intimate way, even to a stranger, to reanimate her.

As a doctor I looked after many patients who were acutely short of breath – with asthma or congestive cardiac failure or advanced lung cancer, for example. Sometimes they were close to choking and I could see the terror in their eyes as they struggled to take each breath. For them, every respiration was literally a matter of life and death. All that mattered was getting in enough air to stay alive. Their relief when medications eased their breathing was palpable.

There is a story from the East that picks up this point. It is about a holy man whose disciple complains of being bored with meditating on his breath. They were sitting by a river. The holy man seized his disciple and pushed his head under the water. No matter how hard the disciple struggled, the holy man would not let go. At last, just when the disciple was about to drown, his master lifted his head out of the water. The disciple gasped, taking in great lungfuls of sweet, life-giving air. "There," said the holy man, "still bored?"

Spirit, then, is the oxygen of the soul. Many years ago I had a dream. I had driven up into the mountains and was travelling along a deserted road. To my left, great mountain peaks covered with snow towered high above me. The rising sun shone brilliantly in the clear, blue sky and the snow was a dazzling white. I saw each plant, each rock, each tree, each stream with a clarity unlike anything I experienced in my waking life. To my right was a slope rising to other heights. The dawn sun shone on the rocks and plants so that they were transformed into a pale radiant gold. I could see the long grasses moving gracefully in the breezes that blew over them. It was entirely beautiful – and ineffable.

My dream, I think, just touched the borders of another world, a spiritual world that interpenetrates our natural world – a sacred way of seeing to which we are mostly blind. There are many, of course, who have had far more intense experiences. They are both blessed and cursed. The Jungian analyst, Robert Johnson (1998), has called this the Golden World, using a phrase coined by Mircea Eliade. A few times in his life he had a vision of such intense beauty that, when he returned to ordinary consciousness, he was desolate and hungered continually over many years to return there.

I remember watching a touching film of cranes, sacred birds, migrating over the Himalayas. In the crisp sunlit morning they slowly circled up on the thermals as they strove in the thin pellucid air to gain enough height to fly over a ridge near the summit of Mount Everest (known as *Chomolungma*, or Holy Mother, by Tibetans). Their demanding journey over such heights was, I thought, a metaphor for our own human spiritual journeys. No wonder so many people try to climb this holy mountain.

Soul Journeys

With Soul, we move to the world of water.

Some years ago, I went turtle watching in Trinidad. Just before darkness we arrived at the beach. It was about five miles long, fringed by coconut trees and deserted. Shortly after night fell, our guides began searching the length of the beach for turtles coming ashore. There was no artificial light and the moon appeared and disappeared as clouds sailed past. It was the sort of natural, deep darkness that you never encounter in a city. After about half an hour, we heard a guide calling. We found a turtle digging a hole for her eggs. She was enormous, a leatherback turtle over six feet long and her eyes wept sticky tears in the unfamiliar air. We could see her tractor tyre tracks emerging from the waves of the ink-black sea. When she started laying her eggs she went into a trance which allowed us turn on our torches without disturbing her; a biologist in the party could take her measurements. Slowly and painfully she began shovelling sand back on to her eighty or so eggs. When she had finished, she levered herself clumsily back into the surf where I knew she would transform into a graceful sea-creature flying in the water as a bird does in the air. I knew her time on land was a tiny fraction of the years she spent at sea.

Our own far distant ancestors came from the sea, primitive sea creatures that gradually evolved lungs to breathe and limbs to move with. No wonder then that we are drawn back to the sea, perhaps to walk by it or to sit on a beach listening to the hypnotic and never-ending rhythm of the waves – our bodies remember where we come from even if our minds do not.

Soul comes from an Old English word *sawol*, meaning the spiritual and emotional part of a person, or animate existence. (Chambers 1988) If, however, you explore this further, you will find that its early German root meaning is 'from the sea'. This is because the sea was considered to be the stopping place of the soul before birth and after death, a curious parallel with our primitive marine ancestors who came ashore much like turtles do now.

There are modern resonances to this story. We spend the first nine months of our life in a womb surrounded by water. Perhaps we re-experience that time of oceanic bliss when we float on the calm waters of a tropical sea, warmed by the sun – or simply have a bath. And, in India, Hindu ritual prescribes that after a cremation the ashes of the dead person are taken and scattered on the sacred waters of the Ganges to be carried down at last to the sea.

Soul, then, is linked with water. It suggests the emotions, fluidity, change and depth; our bodies are more than three-quarters water and, indeed, without it we would die within a few days. Furthermore, the fish, whose element is water, is often used as a symbol for the soul.

However, there is more. There is another soul word, this time from Ancient Greece, namely *Psyche*.

The Search

Nowadays, psyche tends to be used as a synonym for mind, or mental processes. There are, however, different – and deeper – understandings.

In the Louvre in Paris, there is a white marble sculpture called *Psyche Revived by Love's Kiss*, by Antonio Canova. It is an exquisite, tender and erotic work of art. Psyche is naked apart from a cloth draped across the centre of her body. She is lying on her side and Eros has lifted her towards him, his left hand under her right breast and his right hand under the right side of her head. His wings flare upwards behind and above him. He is bringing her lips to his and she, in willing reply, has lifted her arms in a lyre-shaped curve so that her hands touch his head.

What is the story behind this scene? It is one of love, certainly, but also jealousy, tragedy, despair, death and the divine. Psyche is the most beautiful of all mortal women and the god Eros falls in love with her and abducts her to his palace. He only comes to her at night and he never lets her see his face. One night, overcome by curiosity, she lights her lamp and gazes down on the winged god and sees the most beautiful man she has ever set eyes on. It is at this moment that she falls in love with him. She is so overcome by her feelings that the lamp tips and hot oil falls on to the god's skin. He wakes and, wounded by the mortal, scalding oil, flies away crying that she will never see him again.

She searches for him everywhere, desperately and without success. When she appeals to Aphrodite, the mother of Eros, the jealous goddess sets her four impossible tasks, three of which Psyche succeeds in completing.

Finally, in a bid to be rid of her forever, spiteful Aphrodite sends Psyche down into the Underworld, effectively to her death. And Psyche, faithful in her search for her lover, is even prepared to go down into the land of the dead. But this is where

Aphrodite has made her mistake, for it is when Psyche gives up her life for her lover that he, Eros, unable to resist this ultimate sacrifice, comes down to his love and lifts her up to the heavens and eternal life with him. The mortal has become immortal. The human soul has been received into paradise. The statue commemorates Eros reviving Psyche from her deathly trance.

Falling in love, loss and grief, and descent into the Underworld – these three universal human experiences are part of the soul's journey through life and death:

An old, white-haired man sits facing me. I can see he is very anxious. This is our first meeting. Outside the window of the counselling room I can just see trees between the slats of the venetian blinds. It is a day of sun and cloud and the wind insinuates itself through the open window and lifts the blinds slightly so they make a soft scratching sound. I attend carefully as he tells me that his wife died soon after their 45th wedding anniversary. Their marriage had been a very close and loving one. His carefully composed face begins to wobble and tears stream down his face while he struggles to regain control. I remind myself that for older people it often feels shaming to show such emotion in front of someone they do not know. His deep love for his wife is only matched by the profundity of his grief. They were together for most of their lives. How could it be otherwise?

He is a man in his forties, black-haired and sallow-skinned. He has been admitted to a four-bedded bay in a hospice. He sits in bed, his face taut and his staring eyes looking around defensively, and tells me that the nurses are out to get him. He won't take medicines because he believes they are poisoned and is very suspicious of even ordinary nursing care. He seems quite calm as he tells me this. I try first to reason with him but this doesn't work. He is unwilling to believe me. I begin to feel uncomfortable. He is in a psychotic world impervious to everyday logic. He knows he is right. I feel powerless to influence him by persuasion. Later that night he becomes acutely agitated and requires tranquillising drugs to calm him. A couple of days later, when the medicines have controlled his paranoia, he tells me his perception of what happened. The nurses had transmuted into Dutch women wearing traditional hats and dresses. The doctors had become policemen, dressed in black uniforms, peaked hats and guns in holsters. They had come to take him away. It was no wonder he had become agitated. Indeed, he was acting perfectly logically within the confines of the psychotic underworld that was his reality at the time.

Sometimes we act out these descents literally. Ocean explorers descend seven miles under the sea in bathyscaphes. Cavers climb down into the womb-like depths of caves. Adrenaline addicts free-fall from planes or cliffs. Bungee-jumpers bungee-jump off bridges. Would-be suicideers jump off high buildings. LSD users have a bad trip. We bury our dead underground. Sometimes we dream of such descents. Or we watch films or read books in which the action takes place underground or under the sea. Psyche's dark journey in which she repeatedly despairs and then wins through speaks to us all, even when we would rather not listen, because it is something, somewhere in ourselves, that we know.

But there is Paradise, too. There is a famous fifteenth century icon by the Russian painter Andrei Rublev, called, simply, *Trinity*. It is based on the biblical story of Abraham providing hospitality for three angels, who are manifestations of God, by the oak at Mamre. The three figures in the icon are tall and slender with golden wings and long golden curling hair in Byzantine style. They each wear rich robes – gold, wine red, sky blue and spring green. They are grouped around a rectangular altar on which is a chalice containing a small round loaf of bread. Behind them is the oak tree and further back a building, perhaps representing Abraham's tent. The fourth side of the altar is empty and facing the viewer. The intention of the painter is clear – an invitation to join in this sacred meal.

Many years ago, I had a dream about this icon. As I looked at it, I could see that there was a recess in the wall of the altar facing towards me. There was a small door. I stepped forward, opened the door and looked inside. There I saw a small, shining, golden skull.

I have wondered many times about this dream. As I see it now, death, whether of the body or of the ego, is paradoxical. Yes, there is the darkness of loss and dying. But there is another side that promises a transmutation into the gold of a new life. The catch is you may have to walk through a dark valley to get there.

In Ancient Greece, 'psyche' meant both mind and soul. To me, the broader definition makes more sense. We are not just walking adding machines.

Births and Deaths

The first painting has a very simple title: *Le Nouveau-Né* (The Newborn). It is night. There are three figures dressed in peasant clothes current in France over 300 years ago: a young mother, her newborn baby and an attendant. The mother gazes down in rapt silence at her baby who is asleep, wrapped in swaddling clothes, on her lap. Her hands lovingly, carefully and gently support him. Her attendant holds a candle in her left hand, shading it with her right so that a pool of golden light is cast over the three figures making them stand out from the darkness about them. Although it is not immediately obvious, the size of the baby has been subtly magnified as if to emphasise his centrality. It is a picture of utter stillness and, at the same time, complete attention. It was painted by Georges de La Tour between 1645 and 1648 at a time when the Thirty Years War had brought anarchy, murder, plague and famine to his native Lorraine. He didn't call it a nativity, although it clearly is.

The second painting, about 700 years old, is the *Lamentation* by Giotto. Once again Mary is cradling her son on her knees – only now he is dead. Her right arm gently holds his neck and head and her left hand is placed on his chest as if she were hoping she might still feel his heart beating just as she did when he was a child. Her face is contorted with grief. Two women hold his lifeless hands and Mary Magdalene tenderly holds his feet. St John, bent forward, laments, his arms outstretched. Angels rise and fall in the blue sky above joining their anguished weeping with those of the onlookers. A tree on a hill above them reminds us of the Cross.

One of my favourite images showing the cycle of birth and death comes from when I worked at St Christopher's Hospice. (Melville and Schwarz 1990, p. 52) A woman is lying in bed. She is in her fifties and has a strong, smiling face and dark hair. Her daughter is standing by the bed watching her mother and, lying beside the patient, is a newborn baby quietly asleep. You can see the dying grandmother has just been looking at her new granddaughter with such tenderness and pride and now she is looking up at her daughter as if to say: Just look at her. Her daughter could not have given her a better gift.

Rosita and Roberto

A sign on the hospice notice board caught my attention. Rosita and Roberto, flamenco dancers, would be performing that afternoon in the ward dayroom. All were welcome. The invitation was irresistible. I duly turned up.

I found the protagonists preparing for their performance. Roberto was in his late fifties, an Englishman with receding combed-back greying brown hair and a gaunt look. He was dressed in a shirt with ruffles, waistcoat, tight trousers and Mexican heels. His partner, Rosita, about the same age as him, had gone to town on the colourful, layered frills of her dress in which red featured prominently. Her dyed black hair was swept back in a Spanish-style chignon. Heavy make-up accented her eyes; lipstick sang a loud, scarlet song; foundation make-up was much in evidence. A quiet assistant was in charge of the sound system.

Meanwhile, the audience arrived gradually. Many were patients and included one woman wheeled in on her bed.

The great moment arrived and Rosita and Roberto swept on to centre stage. After a brief introduction and a bow, Rosita lifted one curved arm, and, with a flourish of clicks from her castanets, she and her partner launched into their first dance, accompanied by flamenco guitar and singing from their tape. While she gathered her flounces and swung them enthusiastically from side to side, Roberto was strutting his stuff and loudly stamping his heels.

They drew to the end of their dance – and the audience responded with total silence. Unfazed, R and R sprang into action again and, with much brio, flounced and stamped to a new tune. About halfway through, the lady in the bed started to snore. Many would have wilted under this onslaught of inattention, but they stuck to their guns and completed their scheduled presentations exuding the fervour that they obviously felt for flamenco. There was a barely audible ripple of applause at the end to join the continuing snores. I returned to my duties.

Afterwards I wondered why a connection didn't happen. After all, flamenco is a dance about life and barely-contained ardour, and it was probably the wish of most, if not all, in the room that they could go on living rather than die. Maybe, however, at a deep level they knew that they had passed beyond that stage; it was not for them anymore. Even eating and drinking and staying awake were a duty rather than a pleasure. Perhaps they had at some time experienced the passionate engagement with life that flamenco represents. But, that was then and they were now living another season, the time of dying with its own demands.

By contrast, another event I remember in the same dayroom featured old-time songs which brought back memories of the audience's youth. Nostalgic tunes such as *We'll Meet Again* sung by Vera Lynn, or *Lily Marlene*, both from the Second World War, brought an immediate response from those present. Elderly quavering voices joined in, while moist eyes looked inward to the past remembering their part in the war, perhaps the most significant event of their lives and a time when many among them would have cheated death. They loved it.

Many years later, Joan and I went to a flamenco evening presented by Paco Peña, one of the world's leading flamenco guitarists. We had front seats and a close view of the performers. We could even see, as the dancers spun round, the sweat droplets from their hair spiralling out and glittering in the stage lights. They had to be supremely fit to do justice to their extraordinarily demanding dance routines and by the end of each one they were breathing as hard as if they had run a long-distance race. Supporting them were the singers, their bodies shaking with the effort of producing their anguished rough-voiced laments. Here, then, was passion by the bucketful and the audience loved it.

Storms of prolonged applause greeted each number. I could feel the engagement of the spectators in the performance. It spoke to them. Sensual Eros had awoken in their souls. For a little while they were viscerally and passionately alive.

Life has its seasons: a time for passionate life, for remembering, for dying. As long ago as the third century BC, the writers of Ecclesiastes were saying something similar:

> There is a season for everything...: A time for giving birth, a time for dying... a time for healing... A time for tears, a time for laughter; a time for mourning... a time for keeping silent, a time for speaking. A time for loving, a time for hating... a time for peace.
> (The Bible: Ecclesiastes. 3:1–8)

Animals instinctively know such seasons. No one tells them that it is time to migrate, to hibernate or to mate. Their bodies just know what to do. Ours do too if we could but listen, but, being restless humans, we are often estranged from our own natural body rhythms. I think we hanker after this lost inner knowledge and try to recapture it in a thousand different ways, as if it were something that could be grasped and mastered. Actually, it is when we let go and allow our vulnerability that the messages of our body can come through. "I feel sad." "That music is beautiful." "I kept hoping that you would come and visit." "I am so glad to see you." "Just sit with me." Perhaps illness and the threat of death make us to listen afresh to ourselves.

The Fall

It's worth listening to our dreams.

When I was about eight years old, my family and I went on holiday to Belgium and stayed at my grandmother's seaside flat. It was on the sixth floor of a block of flats and overlooked the beach and the sea beyond. It had a long balcony from which we could all watch people passing by on the busy promenade below or on the beach. The lift up to the sixth floor was an ancient rickety affair which swayed as it rose; I sometimes wondered if the cable would break. I loved staying in the flat, the different taste of the food, going down to the beach and swimming. At low tide, the water receded a long way, leaving vast expanses of sand, ribbed by the ebb and flow of the water, and dotted with pale grey, semi-transparent, stranded jellyfish. Sometimes, a group of horses and their riders would trot or canter on the hard, wet sand parallel to the sea. There were huge breakwaters built in a fruitless attempt to prevent the relentless march of sand westward, blown by the prevailing winds. At low tide, these were a wonderful source of crabs, starfish and tiny, greyish, transparent shrimps which we caught with shrimping nets.

My older brother and I shared a bedroom. There was a mosquito net made of fine wire mesh, but there were tears in the mesh which any mosquito worth its salt could easily negotiate. Bites were simply part of the holiday and treated with calamine lotion which dried to a pale fine crust on your skin and then cracked as soon as you moved that part of your body. It was quite satisfying.

One night I had a vivid dream, the most vivid of my childhood. I was standing in a doorway and looking into a ballroom. There were many dancers, the men in white tie and tails and the women in white, lacy bell-shaped ball gowns, swept up hair and diamond necklaces. There were bright chandeliers illuminating the whole room and making the smooth parquet floor glow. The room was a perfect cube and there was a window at the back which showed only blackness. The couples danced in perfect harmony – waltzes, foxtrots and the like. In fact, if Johann Strauss had appeared and conducted one of his Viennese waltzes, he would not have been out of place.

Then I began to fall back. I tried to hold on to the doorway but could not. I fell down and down into utter blackness, while the ballroom receded above me like a dark grey cube spinning in space. As I fell, I was aware of a face to my right, of a dark-haired man with a clipped black beard. He was smiling slightly as he watched me fall. He reminds me now of Mephistopheles, though I don't think I then knew of such a character. I woke to find I had landed on the hard floor by my bed. My heart was beating fast from the fear I still felt from the dream: the terror of falling. But I felt reassured by the solidity of the floor; I could fall no further. I looked out of the meshed window and saw the rays of the pale moon shining in. It felt somehow comforting. The ground held me. My brother remained fast asleep.

In my dream, then, I fell from a place of harmony, a place of grace, down into darkness and the weight of earth's gravity, watched by a shadowy stranger. I was reliving – or perhaps re-dreaming – the mythic story of the Fall of Adam and Eve. This dream still feels poignant to me when I think about it. It is no wonder that this myth still exerts such a fascination for us. It tells a story which has happened to us all, and still does, since myths are outside time.

It was at about that time that I began to experience depression – such a limited word for so intense an experience. It began subtly with times of sadness which even had a certain beauty to them akin to nostalgia. Soon, the black crow gave up all pretensions to attractiveness: instead I felt darkness, heaviness, a grey, cotton wool awareness, numbness, sapped energy, inability to think. Anyone who has experienced depression will know these feelings. It was like walking through life carrying a sack full of stones on my back. Melancholia, that's what Hippocrates would have called it, the old humoral idea of black bile engorging the body with its static excess. He would have briskly prescribed bloodletting to drain the peccant humour. If only.

And yet, there is something important there. Bleeding. Not so much physical as emotional. I know this: when I became sad or frightened, when I grieved or became angry, when my emotions bled, flowed like humours, then I was for a time no longer depressed.

Fighting; that's part of it too. There's a story in Genesis (32:23–32) in which the disgraced Jacob, who has cheated his brother, Esau, out of his heritage, sleeps the night alone by the ford of the river Jabbok. A stranger – a man, an angel, God, who knows – comes upon him and wrestles with him under the wheeling stars all night. And Jacob resists, holds on stubbornly, even when his nameless assailant whacks him so hard that his hip dislocates, till dawn frees him and he limps away to be reconciled with Esau.

It's often hard to tell what's going on inside melancholic people, to sense their dark, fogged distress, their wish to flee from life. But, they're here; they're alive. Somehow they are holding on. It is an interior fight no less heroic for being invisible.

Here's the question: "What heals?" There are people who make dramatic and unexpected recoveries, but I've found it's usually more like putting together the pieces of a jigsaw, one by one, hunting for the right piece, trying several before you find the one that fits, trial and error – a long, patient process.

And the answers I discovered – slowly and painfully – served me in my work with the dying. When patients or family members or clients told me of their distress, of their depression and despair, it has meant that I had a familiarity with what they were talking about. Empathy comes more easily if you have walked a similar path.

Consider this, too: for some people, the thought of falling and falling, seemingly forever, induces utter terror. I know that feeling. I imagine this to be an ancestral memory from our remote forebears who lived in trees. For a newborn to lose purchase of its mother's fur and fall was certain death if not from injury then from the predators that ruled the ground below. I saw this in newborn babies I examined as a doctor. One of the tests I did was called the Moro reflex, named after an Austrian paediatrician called Ernst Moro. When I was taught it, I thought it cruel and developed my own painless, minimalist version. Our teacher would lift a baby, lying on its back in its cot, up by its arms a little and then let go. With this sudden loss of support, the baby's arms would flare out and then come together again and it would cry out from distress. Outstretched arms to hold on to branches; arms coming together to hold on to its mother; crying to alert its mother that her baby was in danger. We are more animal than we know.

We forget that we come from the ground – literally. Our very flesh has been recycled from, what? A blade of grass, a marmoset or perhaps a humpback whale; rich loam or salt licks; an iceberg or the oxygen molecules that their discoverer, Joseph Priestley, once breathed. When, then, we lie down, we ground ourselves, be it on soft sand, pliant grass, hard rock, or a floor of oak planks. Gravity holds us together. If we can tear our treadmill minds away from their endless ruminations, we may find this indescribably comforting. I can fall no further, we may realise. I am held. No wonder the Earth is sometimes called Mother or Gaia.

I work with traumatised people. It takes very little for them to spin back into their dark memories, memories that speed their heart, quicken their breathing, tighten their throat or freeze their very bones. So, no, we do not plunge on regardless and heartless further into their old nightmare. We stop and ground, making a verb of action out of a noun of a place. It is disarmingly literal.

"Just notice your feet on the ground," I say to my client. "No need to change anything, simply notice the sensations of your feet in your shoes (boots, sandals, stilettos, socks, flip-flops, bare feet – it's amazing the variety). Try moving them a little and noticing the sensations changing as you do that." Her attention is shifting to the subtleties of sensation of the skin of her feet. She is coming back into her body and out of the terrifying, mythic Underworld into which she has fallen. Simple. "Notice the chair you're sitting in and how it holds you." So, she can't fall. We turn to her other senses. "What do you hear right now?" I ask. Her attention, previously constricted into a tight tunnel of fear, begins to broaden out. She lets in the wind in the trees, the robin singing, the lawnmower. "Take a look around, what do you see." Her eyes move slowly around, taking in the room, me, the patterned carpet, the soft light from the window, the still books, the pictures. She is here again. "How do you feel?" I ask. "Better," she says. "Calmer." Good.

This is a resource open to all of us.

Life Force

I am repeatedly astonished at the tenacity with which some people cling to life, even if they have, say, an incurable cancer. I first encountered this through my father's work. He was a surgeon and, when I was a child, he would sometimes take me or my brother to the hospital where he practised when he had been called to see a patient. This was back in the 1950s and things were different then. He always wore a formal three-piece suit to work and very shiny round-toed black shoes with laces. Our car was an old, black Ford Prefect. It had a running board and an illuminated orange arrow that flicked out horizontally from its slot in the vertical metal strip between the front and rear windows, when the driver signalled to turn left or right. The leather interior smelt of the cigars he smoked. The hospital, built before the Second World War, was smaller than our modern, multi-storey versions. As we walked along the connecting corridors between low-rise hospital blocks, I could smell the antiseptic hospital smells – methyl salicylate was my favourite. The ward was a large rectangle with space for about thirty beds. It was spotless. The iron beds did not boast any of the modern electronic gadgetry for raising or lowering the head of the bed. They were all neatly made up with starched, white sheets. The patients wore striped pyjamas and, if they were up, brown dressing gowns with spiral piping on the edges. Doctors wore suits, white coats and short-back-and-sides haircuts. Brylcreem was in evidence. The ward sister Sister Hooper was plump, with curly, sandy hair and awesomely efficient. She wore a dark blue uniform and starched apron and cap. She would greet us, in her broad Devon accent, with a bustling smile. I would wait in her office while my father went to see the patient. Often there was a tin of biscuits to sample or old, creased copies of magazines such as *Country Life* to look at. Soon I would hear him return, talking about the patient with Sister Hooper. When their conversation had ended it was time to head home. I always enjoyed these visits. It was as though I was being inducted into another, adult world, a bit like staying up late.

Sometimes he would talk about the patients. When I was a teenager, I remember him telling the story of a woman with advanced ovarian cancer whom he looked after. There was no treatment available and she should have died within a few weeks, at most a few months, he told me. However, he knew that she was determined to live long enough to see her son through school. To her this was of supreme importance. She wanted to support him while he studied so that he had the education necessary to qualify him for finding a career as an adult. My father would see her from time to time and the years passed. Every time he examined her, he noted that the tumour in her abdomen had grown yet larger. Eventually, her whole abdomen was filled with the cancer and yet she hung on. Her son completed his schooling and she died shortly afterwards. When my father told us this story, he would shake his head in disbelief, unable to understand how she had managed to buck the odds for so long. Perhaps hers was an example of the 'fighting spirit' that some researchers have found to increase length of survival.

I was touched by this account, an example of the power of love, and of the life force, the spirit within her that kept her going for as long as was needed. It's not surprising, then, that people with the same cancer and the same staging may differ widely in their length of survival. No wonder, too, that doctors are often so inaccurate in their prognoses of length of survival.

Life Finds a Way

Back in the 1950s my father had a surgical research post in Leeds. We lived in a terraced house in a cobbled street. My father was carrying out research into replacing damaged sections of the aorta, the main artery from the heart down to the legs, with a graft made of Dacron. He tried this out initially with rabbits and a scaled down version of the Dacron tube. He kept some of the rabbits in hutches in our garden. Every day he would tend to their needs, cleaning the hutches out and providing fresh straw, water and food. On one occasion, he had to be away and so he asked my mother to look after the rabbits. The first day she approached the hutches conscientiously and took one rabbit out and put him in with another while she cleaned his hutch. What she didn't realise was that the second rabbit was female. She swore that they were only together for a couple of minutes or so, but during this time, while her back was turned, the rabbits did what rabbits do. By the time she turned back, they were both, I like to imagine, innocently nibbling a quiet post-coital carrot. Unsuspecting, she returned the buck to his hutch. A month later a fine litter of bunnies magically appeared. Clearly, the Dacron graft must have done its stuff since it withstood the rigours of sudden mountainous hikes in blood pressure during the rabbits' covert congress.

Despite the fact that the rabbits had had experimental aortic surgery and that their remaining term of life would be very short indeed, they were not in the least fazed for the simple reason that they had not the slightest idea what was going on. Us humans, however, are cursed with knowledge, knowledge of the present and speculation about the future. Perhaps this is the Tree of the Knowledge of Good and Evil referred to in the Eden story. We might worry that our Dacron graft would burst and we might panic at the thought of dying in short order. Our thoughts revolve around these 'coulds' and fear grows like a dark fruit in these manufactured catastrophic fantasies. Is there anything, then, that we can learn from these 'in the moment' rabbits?

Some people try to live instead in denial even though it's very hard work: true, we can close our eyes to what's happening but unwelcome thoughts and feelings keep popping through our carefully constructed mental barriers. Or we can do the opposite. If you go and visit the Asian gallery at the British Museum, you will find statue after statue of the Buddha and even a beautiful, voluptuous Buddhist goddess called Tara. There is no doubt that they are 'in the moment'. What is striking is the expression of utter stillness on each face, the eyes looking down or closed, a half-smile on each face, their attention withdrawn into the centre of their being. Are they in some faraway dream oblivious of the suffering in the world? Quite the reverse. All four of the Noble Truths that the Buddha taught were about suffering: its existence, its cause, its cessation and the path to freedom from suffering. The message of the statues is very down to earth. The simple act of being aware of fear or despair or pain directly actually makes these dark experiences more bearable. Despite the anxiety that they will continue forever, actually they don't; they rise, plateau and then diminish. They may even go.

At one end of the gallery is a large, stoneware, seated Chinese Buddha called Budai. His enormous belly billows out, shrugging off the folds of his robe. He is not just smiling but laughing and, no doubt, if he could move his belly would be shaking and wobbling in time with his laughter. He has journeyed through suffering, awoken (that is what 'buddha' means) and can't stop laughing about it.

Many years later, I met a patient my father had operated on. He was in his sixties and had been plagued by arterial problems, including an aortic aneurysm (a ballooning and weakening of the wall of the aorta) such that he could hardly walk before his operation. Filled with enthusiasm, he sang my father's praises, smiling all the while. This man had had over the space of several years not one, but three Dacron grafts, one for the aorta and one each for the iliac arteries that carry blood from the aorta down the legs. His life had been transformed; he could now walk easily and normally, and go out. He could not thank my father enough.

I felt very proud of what my father had achieved and I was moved by the patient's story of his transformation. I thought: to have helped another human being who is sick – that surely is something. It was strange, too, that I had been present at the first experimental stages of this operation and then witnessed its fruition.

Extremes

We weren't supposed to go that close according to instructions put up on the notice board of the Visitors' Centre by one of the park rangers. On the other hand Joan and I felt we just could not miss the opportunity.

We are on Big Island which lives up to its name as the largest of the Hawaiian Islands. We have already crossed the huge caldera of Mount Kilauea, a five-mile hike across desolate black lava punctuated by steam venting from cracks in the rock. Far away, to our left, we can see, in the distance, plumes of smoke arising from a sub-vent of Kilauea called Pu'u 'Ō'ō. It has been erupting continuously since 1983. We know that streams of lava flow through underground tubes in the lava fields and then pour into the sea; this can best be seen when it is dark.

That evening, we set off in our car and drive as close as we can to the lava fields. We find an old flow has swept across and obliterated the road. Our plan is to walk across the lava, torches in hand, and get as close as we can to the spectacle. Then a group in a large 4-wheel-drive all-terrain vehicle give us a lift. There is a path of sorts, but it is the roughest ride we have ever experienced. A little way on, we come across a man sitting disconsolately in his car, all four tyres of which have been punctured by the jagged lava. After a quarter of an hour, our driver stops and we all disgorge. He sets up a powerful light on top of his vehicle as a guide to getting back in the dark. We would discover later our need of it. Trekking back across a trackless waste on a dark night with no artificial light, we would find how easy it is to veer away from the car light.

We look around. The sun has just set and we can still see mile upon mile of black volcanic stone, resembling a rough, dark sea frozen in time. It is the bleakest place we have ever seen. We set off, guided by the columns of smoke ahead. Slowly we near our destination. We climb over yet another ridge of lava and see for the first time the origins of the grey clouds rising into the soft, blue evening air. We can make out gouts of semi-liquid red-and-grey lava oozing down from holes in the cliff face, on to a small black beach or directly into the sea. As soon as they hit the water, billowing clouds erupt high in the air. We can smell their intense, sour acidity from where we stand. I have been told it is mostly hydrochloric acid. We watch, mesmerised, as night falls. In the dark, the sight is even more spectacular. There is no daylight to weaken the colours of the molten lava and we can see how its first contact with water makes it explode upwards in a fiery display of intense orange fragments. We are watching new land being created.

In the face of this extraordinary natural power, I feel my littleness. Suddenly, my personal concerns seem insignificant. I will live on this Earth for less than a century; such volcanic eruptions will continue for millions upon millions of years. The overwhelming power of Kilauea dwarfs my frail, vulnerable and short-lived body. When we walked across the caldera, there was a chance that Kilauea could have erupted again at just that spot. No human intervention can stop its future eruptions pouring down over fields, forests and villages, destroying all life as it goes.

And yet I feel excitement too: a sense of awe as we look at this fabulous natural spectacle, and a feeling of sensuous aliveness enhanced by being close to something that could snuff us out in a moment. My body feels energised in synchrony with the power of the vast forces erupting before us.

It seems to me, too, that Kilauea has a life of its own, not in an organic sense but in its fiery mineral power. In traditional Hawaiian mythology, this volcanic life is personified as the beautiful Pele, the goddess of all of Hawaii's volcanoes. She can be both impetuous and violent, and loving and kind. After all, forests and flowering plants grow on her fertile slopes, fed by abundant rains.

Seekers after extreme experiences, such as jumping off the Angel Falls in South America with a tiny parachute to be opened at the last possible moment, will tell you that they feel most alive when they are closest to death. Some dying people say the same.

Breast Is Best

One of the occupational hazards of being a doctor is seeing so many ill people that you begin to think that the world consists only of the sick persons you see and you forget that there are a lot of well people out there. One might say that liver specialists, for example, have a jaundiced view of life. Surgeons might size up fellow passengers travelling in the Tube for operations. Cardiologists walking down the street would be on the lookout for people at risk of cardiac disease – the driven executive, the smokers or the overweight or all three together. Oncologists would notice those with suspicious swellings and wonder about their diagnosis.

And palliative medicine specialists such as myself? I can't help noticing those with advanced incurable illnesses. I remember once going to a parents' meeting at my son's school. There was a man walking slowly along accompanied by his wife and son. The man's face was pale and slightly jaundiced. His hair was all but gone. His abdomen protruded. He breathed heavily as he walked. I knew immediately that he was dying, almost certainly from advanced cancer. I had seen many people just like him in my work. My heart went out to him and his family. I admired his courage in making a huge effort to attend the meeting for his son's sake. I hoped that he would respond to whatever palliative treatment he might be taking and would live long enough for them to say their goodbyes.

Palliative medicine is particularly difficult from this point of view since, in the end, it is always about dying. I have needed to keep reminding myself that everyday life away from work does not revolve only around death. The same applies when I examine patients. I suppose I have seen many hundreds of women who have had a mastectomy for breast cancer. I need to bear in mind that, actually, the majority of women have not had this operation.

I remember an occasion when this was vividly brought home to me. I was on holiday in Brittany with my family. We were visiting a little seaside town and in the morning went down to the beach. There was a stone wall about ten feet high with steps leading down from the road to the sand. Nearby there was a small group of Breton youth standing by the wall to our left. There was an intensity about them. They shifted around uneasily and talked quietly to each other. The cause soon became apparent. To our right a mother and daughter were sunbathing. After a while, the daughter, who could not have been more than eighteen years old, got up to have a relaxing stroll. She was topless and her bikini bottom was about as brief as it could be while still maintaining its concealing function. As if by chance, she headed out past where the Breton youth were standing. Her hair fell in a loose mane and her skin was a beautiful, soft, amber colour. Her breasts were perfect and seemed to have some invisible means of support allowing them to sway gently as she walked. Every now and then she artlessly dragged a toe in the sand and then, as if spontaneously, she stretched her flexed arms back and took a deep breath so that her breasts swayed forwards and her nipples jutted yet more obviously in best Mills and Boon fashion. The Breton youth were transfixed. An invisible miasma of lust surrounded them. They pretended not to look, but eyes darted shiftily sideways to ensure they missed nothing.

Having reached the end of her tiring walk, she turned around and reprised her performance – toe dragging, stretching, nipple jutting – as she headed back to her beach towel. She had them in the palm of her hand. It was a bravura performance. It wasn't designed to initiate a long-term relationship of course, but then that wasn't the point. She was revelling in the power of her sexuality and the spellbinding effect of her beautiful breasts on the hapless youths with whom she toyed.

And for me, it was a transition point. A few days before, at work, I had been seeing older women ill from breast cancer. Here, on holiday, I had, as it were, gone back fifty or sixty years to a time when these elderly women had been just like this beautiful, healthy teenager with her beautiful, healthy breasts. An important reminder.

Chapter 3

Roots

Opposite the Science Museum in Exhibition Road in London is a white, spired building, the Church of the Latter-Day Saints. If you go inside and turn several corners, you will find stairs leading to the basement. Follow these down and you will come to a series of linked rooms filled with computers and microfilm readers. The rooms are packed. A crowd of people sit studying the images they have called up on these machines: three hundred year old parish registries of births, deaths and marriages; nineteenth century passenger lists on ships bound for the colonies; convict lists from Australia; eighteenth century wills; property transactions; coats of arms; army records; old newspapers. This sight, more than anything else, brings home to me how important our past is to us, for our ancestors are our roots. True, some may have been adulterers, bigamists, murderers or convicts, but we exist only because they existed.

Sometimes, we want to forget our past. We have experienced pain, rejection or failure, and would rather these memories were permanently erased from our consciousness, buried in some deep underground chamber and the key thrown away. Would that it were so simple. As the philosopher Santayana (1905, p. 284) said, "Those who cannot remember the past are condemned to repeat it." Of course it doesn't help to rehearse distressing memories from the past endlessly. That way they may feed on each other and grow, a sort of emotional malignancy. But if we think of re-membering the past, we make it a member of our being. We give these memories meaning. They become part of who we are.

The Healing Tree

When I find the press of city life, of crowds, noise and traffic, too much I sometimes go out into the country to visit a tree I know. Actually it is one of a pair of tall beech trees with massive trunks and spreading branches. Beech mast litters the ground around the trees along with a few overladen branches which have broken off in high winds. Roots plunge deep into the earth leaving hollows between them that make convenient, if rather uncomfortable, seats. In the cold seasons, they are covered with bright green moss fed by the winter rains. The bark is quite smooth with a pale greenish-grey colour. Above is a thick canopy of soft green leaves, a good shelter from the rain.

I enjoy just sitting in one of the hollows between the roots and sensing the solidity and the immense strength of the tree. It feels comforting and calming, a refuge from our driven collective busyness. From there, as I eat my lunch, I can look over a vista of fields, variegated woodland and streams, and watch and listen to the woodpigeons, green woodpeckers and the occasional pheasant go about their avian affairs. It's a wonderful restorative for nerves keyed up by the feeling of too much. I feel more centred and, literally, more grounded.

Trees, however, are not just trees. They are also important players in our mythic world. The Garden of Eden boasted two wonderful archetypal trees – the Tree of the Knowledge of Good and Evil, and the Tree of Life. In the middle of our first paradisiacal home, a place outside time, are these two arboreal symbols, whose fruits confer wisdom and immortality. We all know what happened when Adam and Eve, tempted by the subtle serpent, took a bite each from the forbidden fruit of the wisdom tree – exile, hardship, pain and death.

But the other tree, the Tree of Life, is hardly mentioned. And yet, what a tree! One that gives life, confers immortality. Isn't this what we all long for? don't we all wish to feel alive, intensely alive? If we are seriously ill, don't we search anxiously for the elixir that will heal us? CS Lewis wrote about this in *The Magician's Nephew* (1963), one of the famous Narnia fantasy series he penned for children. In the book, Digory and Polly magically travel from Victorian London to Narnia at the very moment when it is being created by the lion, Aslan. Digory must bring Aslan an apple from a tree in a walled garden at the top of a green hill in the middle of a blue lake surrounded by high ice mountains. It is the Tree of Life and its seeds are to grow into a tree protecting Narnia from evil. This task is doubly hard for Digory because, back in London, his mother is dying and he longs to bring her a silver Apple of Life to heal her. He resists the almost overwhelming temptation to run away from his task and return to her with a stolen apple. Instead he brings the fruit to Aslan and it is planted. It seems his opportunity has gone. But the tree grows fast in this new world, still infused with the creation song the lion sang, and Digory is permitted take an apple from this new tree and return to his mother.

The scene where Digory tenderly feeds his mother slices of the apple and watches her recover is moving enough but it is even more so if we know that the author's own mother died of cancer when he was ten years old and that when she was ill he used to bring her gifts that he hoped would make her better. When she died, he was distracted with grief; his desperate prayers for her cure had not been answered. His happiness withered. So, when, years later, he wrote about Digory's quest, he was speaking from the deep pain of his own experience of loss. (Arnott 1983)

There are many stories in traditional cultures around the world about sacred trees. This is not surprising when you consider that their roots are anchored in the earth and their upmost branches reach up to heavens. In mythic terms, then, trees unite Heaven and Earth – of course they are sacred. It is curious, in this context, how we humans describe our minds as having the same three levels: we speak of a subconscious which we equate with the subterranean world; consciousness which is our present moment awareness as we stand on the surface of the Earth; and a superconscious where we receive intimations of the divine.

Trees play their part in religions, too. The Buddha became enlightened under a Bodhi tree – perhaps another wisdom tree? In the moonlit Garden of Gethsemane, a grove of ancient olive trees witnessed Jesus' anguished prayer to be spared his fate – and it was to a tree that he was nailed the next day.

Trees do literally show an extraordinary tenacity to life, and I am not just talking about recovering from their annual loss of leaves in winter. In a park where I go walking, there is the trunk of a large horse chestnut tree which has been cut down. Its branches have been amputated; nothing could be more dead you would have thought. But around the stump of the tree are growing thirty or more shoots, each producing the characteristic five-fingered leaves of chestnut trees. Along the trunk, one of the stumps of the amputated branches is buried in the ground. Above it, growing from the joint of the branch with the trunk are more leaved shoots. Just by it, shoots grow out of the ground. The stump of the branch has, against the odds, taken root. It lives on. I feel like cheering whenever I pass it by.

Our very lives, of course, depend on trees. Apart from being the lungs of the Earth, they can, of themselves, bring life to barren places. One of my favourite books is called *The Man Who Planted Trees* by Jean Giono (1954). In it, the writer is walking in the desolate mountainous region between Provence and the Alps. There is little water and the villages are abandoned. He meets a shepherd, Elzeard Bouffier and stays at his cottage. He discovers that the shepherd has been systematically planting acorns for years; ten thousand have taken root and produced shoots so far. Over decades the writer returns on several occasions and, bit by bit, he watches the growth of great swathes of trees spread over many kilometres, from tiny saplings to strong young trees. With the trees, water returns and brooks run again; at last people return to the abandoned villages he had passed through. He visits one and sees how they have rebuilt the ruined houses and church, and constructed a fountain in the square for drinking water. Now they can grow vegetables and fruit in their gardens and farm the land around the village. Life has returned to the once desolate land.

Some people don't change much after a bout with cancer. They go back to life as it was before their illness. Some, however, change radically. They may describe their life before cancer as empty and meaningless – indeed as a desolate land. Somehow their encounter with cancer puts them in touch with a different reality. Their priorities change.

It is as though their inner landscape has been transformed – formerly a desert, it has come to life. But this is a soulscape, a mythic place where everything is more than it seems. Here, the Tree of Life can flourish again. How strange that all this should come about through such a dreaded illness as cancer.

The Cave

When I was at school, I used to go caving and potholing in the
Mendip Hills in Somerset, especially in the Cheddar Gorge. I
remember the mixture of excitement and apprehension I felt as
my companions and I peered down into the blackness of a cave's
entrance, knowing the tunnel descended far into the dark depths
below us. Caves, I learned, were classed as wet or dry. Wet meant
there was a stream running through them. Dry, however, did not
necessarily mean dry at all. All manner of seepages through
cracks in the limestone rock and of pools to be negotiated
conspired to make us almost as soaked as in a wet cave. I
remember the sharp, cold, damp, mineral smell of the caves and
the tart odour of our acetylene lamps attached to our blue
helmets. Without their light we would be plunged in absolute
darkness. Then there were the tight squeezes to wriggle through,
too tight for comfort sometimes. Some of the other boys spoke of
their anxiety at having millions of tons of rock bearing down on
them, though for some reason this never troubled me. I do recall,
however, my uneasiness about getting lost in the underground
labyrinth that most caves are.

Caves are a potent symbol for the primeval aspects of our
collective and individual unconscious. The earliest humans
would have used caves for shelter and safety. Deep inside they
painted sacred images of their world, of the animals they hunted
and of their shamans. Caves were dangerous, too. Predators such
as bears lived in them. It is easy to imagine how such animals
might have been the origins of terrifying mythical beasts that
lived deep beneath the earth. "Here be dragons", as the old maps
might say, dragons that liked nothing better than to lie greedily
on their vast, stolen cache of treasure in an underground hall.
And Tartarus, the place in Ancient Greek mythology where the
dead went, was also called the Underworld. Caves inhabited by

early humans or Neanderthals have been discovered containing skeletons buried there. The dead were literally underneath the living.

I remember a conversation I had with one man who had been successfully treated for cancer. He told me of an image that had come to him spontaneously. It seemed to him that his psyche was like a mineshaft – an artificial cave – that went deep underground; many side tunnels branched off at many different levels, each representing an aspect of his unconscious being. As he talked, I had a sense of the hugeness of this place in his imagination. It felt as if we had explored a little of this vast network, but far more remained, waiting for the light of his awareness to plumb its depths, the work of a lifetime perhaps.

An Immortality of Hands

In Chauvet cave in Southern France, a treasure trove of 35,000 year old rock paintings, there is one image I find particularly moving (Clottes 2003, p. 84). It is a hand stencil, made by the artist placing his right hand with spread fingers against the rock and blowing red ochre powder on to it – a sort of visual signature perhaps. One can see that his thumb is misshapen and that he holds his third and fourth fingers close together. Perhaps these are old hunting injuries. The image could have been made yesterday and yet it is six times as old as the pyramids. As I look at this ancient handprint, I feel a sort of vertigo as if the gap between then and now has momentarily slipped and he is nearby, in the next room – or cave chamber. Linear time has become a spiral, and looped back on itself. He and I are, after all, one species. Perhaps his DNA has contributed through many thousands of generations to mine.

We fear extinction, fear disappearing absolutely leaving no trace, as if we never existed. No wonder we try to leave our mark; no wonder we research our ancestry to keep alive our origins. And yet, this simple hand silhouette felt more significant to me than the monoliths left by powerful rulers trying to ensure a privileged place in the afterlife such as the immense tomb of the first emperor of China, guarded by an impotent terracotta army that had disintegrated into pottery shards when it was excavated.

Some people close to death begin a memory box to leave to their children and grandchildren, containing memorabilia of significant events in their life – photos, postcards, poems, pictures, lockets of hair, tickets to special events, a diary from childhood, a diary of that person's thoughts during her last illness, and natural objects such as shells, stones or feathers which hold a special family meaning. There might even be brooches, bracelets, gold chains or rings with instructions as to who is to inherit them.

My father passed on to me a beautifully machined brass microscope which he had used during his medical training in the 1930s in Australia. It had its own mahogany box with sliding wooden inserts to hold the various eyepieces. The microscope fitted into slots in the box perfectly and there were velvet pads to prevent damage during transit. Inscribed on to the base of the microscope was the name of the manufacturer, *E. Leitz Wetzlar*. Somehow, this German-made microscope had found its way out to Australia. On the floor of the box my father had written his name and address in Sydney, Australia, in faded brown ink. There was a bottle of immersion oil and a box of microscope slides which had been made in Belgium. A chamois leather hood protected the upper part of the microscope. Its smell was an evocative mixture of metal, wood and oil. I would guess it to be a century old by now. I think he gave it to me because he knew I was interested in natural history, but I believe, too, he was bequeathing something of his vocation to me. For me, it is redolent of the past; I can still see him sitting at his desk and talking to me about the microscope and its workings. It is a link for me with him and his life in Australia, with another age and another place. Hands played a part here, too, since when he handed it to me, it was into my hands. For a moment I imagine an endless chain of hands down the generations before me and after me. If we can have an exultation of larks and a pod of whales, why not an immortality of hands?

Ancestral Lines

A person's family and ancestry can say much about him.

Joan and I were on holiday and driving down a long wooded sloping valley that led to Sedona in Arizona. On the edge of the city we saw a sign saying: Trading Station. Curious, we drove up the short dirt track to a building which looked like the sort of cabin pioneers used to construct. There was a fence made of round poles – just the sort to which cowboys would nonchalantly tie the reins of their horse in innumerable Westerns. On another fence was draped a huge brindled bull's hide – from South America I later discovered. We went in.

The owner, bearded and longhaired, sat behind a wooden counter where there were postcards of early photographs of Native Americans. One caught our eye because we had seen it in England. Taken in 1898, it shows a beautiful eight year old Native American girl called Katie Roubideaux Blue Thunder. Behind her is a featureless backdrop such as photographers used then. She is wearing a long, tasselled deerskin shift meticulously embroidered with complex beaded patterns, as are her leggings and moccasins and the floor covering on which she stands. She is holding a doll in the crook of her left arm. Her head is shyly inclined to her left so that that side of her face is in shadow.

We began to explore the building. To our left was a series of rooms containing a multitude of Indian artefacts – tomahawks, arrows, arrowheads, bows, knives, bowls, fossil shells and so on. These were made by local Native Americans mostly for the tourists. Here and there I spotted an insignificant-looking, quite dull object such as a bowl made from woven cord. These retailed for three or four times the price of other much showier bowls; they were genuine Indian artefacts, some 50 or 100 years old.

On the right were more rooms which were very different. For a start, they had several animal skins. One was of a cougar and I could see the two bullet holes at chest level from the rifle that killed it. There was a long dresser with an array of small drawers such as one might use to hold buttons. Their contents were, however, very different. There were chicken claws, bear teeth, semi-precious stones, feathers from various birds such as crows and eagles, a huge variety of animal bones, preserved animal paws, and so on. On the walls were the skulls of animals such as deer and cattle. I was fascinated. Paradoxically I also felt I wanted to back away. I was in the presence of the remains of many dead animals. There is no equivalent that I know of in England. Shops in Britain are sanitised and safe, purveying inanimate items made of plastic, rubber, glass or metal. Even supermarkets pre-prepare meat and fish, wrapping them in cling-film. The trading station was very different. I felt a powerful, concentrated energy there; it was like whisky in comparison to the watered-down beer of shopping malls. Furthermore, these items were not particularly aimed at tourists. Many could only have been, I thought, for Native American religious rituals.

A little earlier, Joan had been in the entrance room and had seen a middle-aged mixed race Native American, with the sort of moustache that Sheriff Pat Garrett had sported during his conflict with Billy the Kid, come in, talk to the owner and then leave. Later, as we made our purchases and looked again at the postcard of the little girl, he told us that the man who had just been in was her grandson. He was a tribal healer or shaman and was visiting Sedona. His grandmother had lived to the age of 101 and died in 1991. Her father had been an interpreter for a Sioux reservation and in the Indian police.

I was struck by this synchronicity and by the way that the past and present had fortuitously collided for us in this trading station. I wondered what it was like for her to live in a climate of confinement and of subjugation, where one race proclaimed itself superior to the other. What was it like to be mixed race, yet not accepted by white people who shared some of her genetic heritage? It seemed appropriate that her grandson had become a healer. Healing, while it takes place in the present, is often about the past reaching back down the ancestral lines of each person. Humanity's crimes against itself such as the treatment of Native Americans by white settlers, the Slave Trade or the Holocaust cast a shadow down future generations, both of oppressors and oppressed. Sometimes, people are born whose life purpose seems to be to bring healing to themselves, to their family and even to their tribe, culture or race.

The Ship and the Tree

"My name is Violet," said Violet, our guide during our walk in the Australian rainforest. Stocky and good-humoured, she let us know she was mixed Aborigine and white, and proud of her heritage. I liked her direct way of facing an issue that Australia still has not resolved. We set off. I used to imagine that a rainforest was so stuffed full of vegetation of the Swiss cheese plant variety that you had to hack your way through it inch by inch, plying your razor-sharp machete. Not so this one. From the path it was quite easy to see some distance through the undergrowth in the greenish light filtering down through the canopy.

Violet showed us points of interest: a beautiful forest iguana clinging motionless to a tree trunk, a traditional bark shelter, edible plants, other medicinal plants, a leaf that could be used as soap, tendrils used as string, stones used to make paints, the women's pool (I had to retreat until I was out of earshot so that Violet could instruct Joan in the secrets of this place). There were, however, two places she took us to which particularly struck me. One was a rock face with Aboriginal paintings on it. There were an emu, a stingray, a turtle and a shaman dancing. One image, though, was of a ship, a strange ship with a long bowsprit, a series of black dots along its side, a mast with a square object at the top and a diagonal line above. The sails were not the usual sharp triangles. They ballooned out so that the edge of each sail formed a wide semicircle.

"Now this is Captain Cook's ship," said Violet nonchalantly. I stared at her and then again at the image, amazed. The blob at the top of the mast must be the crow's nest, I thought, and the strange round sails an attempted portrayal of the square European sails of the 18th century by an artist unfamiliar with them and the way they caught the wind giving the effect of curved edges. The diagonal line above the crow's nest was a flag. The black dots on

the side of the ship were portholes for the cannons. I was fascinated.

Captain Cook had dropped anchor not far from here in 1770
when his ship, the Endeavour, was badly damaged by a coral
reef – part of the Great Barrier Reef – while he was charting the
East Coast of Australia. The seven weeks needed for repairs
would have given the local Aborigines plenty of time to study
the strange vessel.

It seemed such an innocent picture of a herald from across the
seas, but, from my present vantage point 240 years later, it was
all too easy to see its shadow side; it was a portent of the future
when the indigenous Aboriginal peoples were almost swept
away by a vast tide of European immigration. As a doctor I think
especially of the devastating effects of illnesses that were
brought in by such ships. Thus, within a year of the foundation
of the first penal colony in Sydney in 1789, local Aborigines were
all but wiped out by smallpox, a disease to which they had no
natural immunity. Here is a contemporary account of the grief of
Arbanoo, a captured Aborigine, when he saw the devastation
wrought among his people: "He lifted up his hands and eyes in
silent agony for some time; at last he exclaimed, 'All dead! All
dead!' And then hung his head in mournful silence." (Barwick
1998, p. 296)

The other place that Violet took us to was a tree, a strangler
fig to be precise. It was one of the strangest trees I have ever seen.
The trunk was an interlaced pattern of slim, vertical, sinuous
trunks, each about the diameter of a didgeridoo, some thicker,
some thinner, many partially fused together. Through the gaps
we could see that the twisting knotted trunks left a wide hollow
in the centre, twenty feet across and open to the sky. The tree rose
to a height of well over a hundred feet. Arthur Rackham would
have loved to draw it. It had that mythic otherworldly quality
found in fairy tales and myths that he captured so well in his
pictures. He might have called it Old Man Tree and endowed it

with a beard, human intelligence and speech: full of wisdom but not to be trifled with.

Violet explained: the strangler fig started life as shoots like an ivy. They would climb a tree, spreading and diverging, gaining in strength all the time, wrapping the tree in their many-fingered branches as if they were boa constrictors. Gradually the supple shoots became woody trunks which slowly strangled their host. When the tree died it rotted away, leaving the fig now able to stand by itself.

This was a sacred tree for the local Aborigines, Violet told us, and its hollow heart was still used for their religious ceremonies. I could imagine it. Tall and old, it had a cathedral-like quality. It inspired respect. We instinctively lowered our voices while we looked at it. I asked if we might take photographs. "Yes," she said. "Because I'm here. But don't go inside the tree." The unspoken message was clear. If we lacked respect we might run into trouble. This tree was not just an arboreal species; it was at the same time a powerful Dreaming spirit not to be trifled with.

But there was something else. Despite the tide of destruction that the Aboriginal nation had experienced, it had survived, and this tree, a focus of their religious expression, was an example. It was strange to find the juxtaposition of Captain Cook's ship, a harbinger of calamity, and this tree, a sign of hope, all within the space of an hour.

As we walked back to our starting point for tea and damper, I looked at Violet. She was both Aboriginal and White. She believed in both her Aboriginal religious traditions – the Dreaming ancestors – and, at the same time, in Jesus – she showed us the large cross she was wearing. Here was one person embodying in her own way rapprochement, healing and forgiveness.

The Jar of Opium

I have two old pharmaceutical jars, shaped like short-necked goblets, which I inherited when my mother died. They are delftware, made of pottery and coarsely glazed so that spots of the clay come through. The background is white and beginning to craze. Each has an inscription in blue lettering. One says EX JUNIPER. The other says LAUD:OP:B:F. These are surrounded by a roughly-painted crest with two peacocks above the writing and a small winged cherub's face below, as if it were holding up the crest. In the second jar I can see a greyish, powdery remnant stuck to the bottom of the pot.

Extract of juniper doesn't figure in pharmacies nowadays, but, unbelievably, laudanum does, although now it's known as tincture of opium. I am intrigued that there is still a dusting of what I take to be the opium from which it was made still in the jar. To me, this is a happy coincidence, since morphine, an extract of opium, has been one of the main pain relieving drugs I have used in palliative medicine. Just as with us humans, its story deserves investigation.

We tend to think of the conquest of pain in terms of general anaesthetics brought into use in the 19th century, with a dark age of endless suffering stretching back through time. The truth is not so simple. The first written record of opium being used was about 5000 years ago in what is now Iraq. They called it the joy plant – for obvious reasons. This means that one of the most powerful analgesics known to humanity has been available, and used, to relieve suffering for millennia, quite how long nobody knows. Present day indigenous peoples living traditionally are extraordinarily knowledgeable about the medicinal properties of forest plants and adept at using them. It's reasonable to assume, then, that early hunter-gatherers, with their innate human curiosity, would have been aware of the properties of the opium poppy tens of thousands of years ago. Every time, then, that I have prescribed morphine or another similar opioid, I have been following in the footsteps of the countless thousands of physicians and healers and tribal shamans in the past who relieved suffering with some form of extract from the opium poppy.

The 17th century English physician, Thomas Sydenham, who concocted his own version of laudanum by mixing opium with sherry-wine, saffron, cinnamon and cloves – it was a runaway bestseller – made the following enthusiastic observation: "And here I cannot but break out in praise of the great God, the Giver of all good things, who hath granted to the human race, as a comfort in their afflictions, no medicine of the value of opium." (Sydenham 1848, p. 173) I have lost count of the many times I have confirmed how true that statement is. Here is one example:

I was working as a registrar, in training at St Joseph's Hospice in 1979. I had been seconded to the Home Care Team and I was called out to see a patient with advanced cancer at home who had suddenly developed severe pain. It was late afternoon when I arrived and the winter day was drawing to a close when I parked near her second floor flat. I rang the bell and, as soon as the door was opened by the woman's husband, it was obvious that she was in crisis – I could hear her groaning even from the entrance hall. Their parish priest was sitting with her as I entered the brightly lit bedroom, a contrast to the darker hallway. She was restless, breathing fast, moaning, pale, her lips blue, her face drawn in agony. Examining her, her rigid abdomen was acutely tender. I have rarely seen a person in such distress. I thought she had perforated her bowel. She was not going to live long. However, I had the impression, which I have often seen, that the severity of the pain was actually preventing her from letting go into her dying. It was like a dark fist that had grabbed hold of her, and her body had responded as if it were under attack. Massive surges of adrenaline had poured through her body. Her restlessness was her instinctual desire to escape but she could not because any movement of her abdomen worsened her already intense pain.

The contrast after I had given her an injection of diamorphine and tranquillisers was extraordinary. Her rapid breathing gradually calmed, her previously speedy pulse slowed to a normal rate, her moaning stopped, her limbs ceased their restless movements, the tense lines on her face smoothed out and she drifted into sleep. We sat with her as she lay quietly in the bed, breathing slowly and regularly. With the pain relieved, her body could relax. Escape in a storm of adrenaline was no longer needed. Now she could let go. The fist had released its grip. For a while she remained the same, balanced between life and death. Some time later, her breathing slowed, then stopped. She had died, free of pain. It was a privilege to sit with her during her passing.

I am glad that I was able to relieve her suffering, just as I have been on many similar occasions over the years. What could be more helpful to someone in such straits? And it began with the opium poppy; it began with the first person, time out of mind, to cut into the head of the poppy, taste its sap, and discover its magical properties: not only euphoria but also relief from pain. And this knowledge was passed down, generation after generation. My opium jar is really a latecomer on the scene, a mere couple of centuries old. The dawn of humanity is a much-overused phrase. Still, in this case, there may be some truth in saying it reaches back to such a time.

Chapter 4

Wounding

We have all had some kind of a physical wound, whether this was a minor scratch or major trauma from a car accident. We know what wounds are with their disruption of the skin which covers us, revealing the bleeding flesh underneath. What is less easy to imagine are wounds of the psyche, wounds to the soul. There is no splitting of visible matter here, no loss of blood; nonetheless we feel such injuries acutely, we feel our integrity has been disrupted and, unlike flesh wounds, their effect may continue unabated over decades.

I remember hearing the story of a teacher who survived the First World War, albeit with what was then called shell shock. He returned to his job. His pupils, with the casual cruelty of some adolescents, used to imitate the whistling of a bomb falling. He was unable to stop himself from diving under the table where he cowered terrified while his pupils sniggered, exulting in their power over him. That painful legacy would stay with him for many years, since no effective treatments were then available for such trauma.

It's important to remember that such wounds are just as real as physical ones. Actually, they do have a visibility, though in a different way to physical injuries.

The Greek myths, with their soulful nature, can help us here. Thus, there is the story of Medusa, a hideous Gorgon with coiling serpents for hair, whose stare was so terrifying that it turned people to stone. Traumatised people may become frozen, hardly able to move, pale, speechless, their eyes staring – in effect, turned to stone.

Then there is the legend of Sisyphus, condemned by Zeus to roll a boulder eternally to the top of a hill only to have it roll back down again. He was helpless to prevent this happening and had to start all over again. One of the major symptoms of the injured psyche is that of feeling overwhelmed and helpless.

There is also the Titan, Prometheus, who stole fire from the gods to give to humanity. Zeus punished him by having him chained to a rock. Each day an eagle would come and tear out the Titan's liver. Every night it would regenerate and the eagle would return the next day to reprise its gruesome task. Traumatic memories have a habit of returning again and again whether in flashbacks or nightmares.

Oedipus, the newborn son of King Laius and Queen Jocasta of Thebes, was exposed on a mountainside and left to die because of a prophecy that he would kill his father and marry his mother. Children experience abandonment in a thousand ways: they may be left in their room to cry; they may be ignored and rejected by their parents who favour another sibling; their parents may be emotionally unavailable to them; they may be sent to boarding school; they may be put in care.

And there is Persephone, the beautiful daughter of Zeus and Demeter, the harvest goddess. With Zeus' connivance, his brother Hades, god of the Underworld, abducted and raped Persephone, forcing her to be his queen. Here, then, are the twin themes of rape and incest, both of which take place in the shadowlands of our present society.

The truth is that just about all of us have received some kind of traumatic wounding in our lives.

Soul Work

His father died when he was seven, his tubercular mother when he was fifteen. His brother died of the same illness when he was 25. His poetry was savagely attacked by critics, though now he is one of the most famous and well-loved English poets. He had an unhappy love affair and died of tuberculosis in Rome aged 25. John Keats, who studied medicine, died young after much suffering. He was not, however, embittered by his struggle. In a journal letter, written the year he died, to his brother and sister, George and Georgiana, Keats wrote:

> I will call the world a School Book used in that School and I will call the Child able to read, the Soul made from that School and its hornbook. Do you not see how necessary a World of Pains and troubles is to school Intelligence and make it a Soul? A place where the heart must feel and suffer in a thousand diverse ways!... As various as the Lives of Men are so various become their Souls, and thus does God make individual beings, Souls...
> (Scott 2002, p. 291)

He coined the phrase, the "Vale of Soul-making" (Scott 2002, p. 290) to describe his idea that the soul matures during its journey through life with all its vicissitudes.

Tom was about four years old when he was admitted to the paediatric ward where I was working. He was the only son of older parents – they were in their late forties – who doted on him. They had almost given up hope of having a child when he came along. At first it seemed like a straightforward case of croup, but during the day he rapidly deteriorated. The infection was affecting his trachea and lungs as well as his larynx. His breathing became increasingly laboured, his chest heaving, his skin colour pale blue. He was put in a steam tent with oxygen. My consultant came in to see him. Tom was close to needing artificial ventilation. His parents were in shock, staring helplessly at their beloved child, in agony at seeing him so distressed. I had the uneasy feeling that Tom's illness was spiralling out of control. However, as I was listening to the deliberations of the other doctors involved in his case, I noticed something out of the corner of my eye. Whenever Tom was asked to cooperate with the nurses in moving him, and with the physiotherapist in helping him to clear his chest secretions and to breathe more efficiently, he actively tried to assist them, even though he himself could hardly move from breathlessness and was obviously very frightened. I was touched by the courage and tenacity of this small boy. I thought that few four year olds would have been able to do what he was doing.

For another couple of days, his condition hung in the balance and then, very slowly, he began to improve. His breathing was a little less difficult, his colour less grey. His recovery accelerated, as is the way with children, and within a few days he was back to his usual self, energetic, cheerful and playing with the other children on the ward.

What helped him through this crisis? Firstly, it was clear his very loving parents had brought him up to have a basic trust in other people – quite an achievement. Secondly, his illness called out of Tom the courage to face his crisis. We could say that this courage had always been there as a potential ready to be released when the occasion demanded. Michelangelo once said that the sculpture he was working on was already there in the marble. His job was simply to chip away the redundant stone to reveal what had been present all along. Perhaps it is the same with the soul.

A Quartet of Pains

As part of my training in palliative medicine, I worked for a couple of years at St Christopher's Hospice, which had been founded by Dame Cicely Saunders. Her work was the catalyst which has led to the spectacular development of the modern hospice movement.

I used to watch her when she gave a lecture or took part in the weekly Grand Rounds on the wards. She was tall, stooped and grey-haired and always reminded me of a dowager duchess. She wouldn't have been out of place in a PG Wodehouse novel. Her eyes had a hawk-like piercing quality. She had, too, a sharp, sometimes fierce intelligence, which belied the deep compassion she felt for the dying in her care. This combination of an incisive intellect and an empathy for those with life-threatening illnesses drove her in her quest to found St Christopher's, with its emphasis on the best of multidisciplinary clinical care and research. It took her 19 years; such dogged persistence.

Again and again, peering at us challengingly over her half-moon glasses, she would, like a mantra, come back to her concept of *Total Pain*, comprising physical, psychological, social and spiritual elements, all of which interacted with each other. This model could, of course, be applied just as well to any illness. It seemed so obvious: pay attention not only to the body, but also to the mind, relationships and soul. It was indeed whole person care. She would remind us that each part must be given attention if a dying person's suffering was to be effectively relieved. Did we want to know why a patient's physical pain wasn't responding to analgesics? It might be because we had missed his unresolved grief following the death of his wife a year before. And if another patient was intractably anxious, was there a simmering feud in his family? Perhaps what we took to be a straightforward diagnosis of depression might actually mask spiritual distress, what St John of the Cross so vividly called the dark night of the soul. It was a simple but highly effective approach. It was also quietly revolutionary. She was, as far as I know, the first doctor in the 20th century deliberately to include all four areas in the mainstream medical care of the dying. Perhaps this was because her previous training as a nurse and then a social worker had enabled her to see ill people from several viewpoints at once, all of them important.

Splits

Modern medicine retains some strange throwbacks to its distant past. One of these is the Staff of Asklepios. Ancient Greek statues show the divine physician carrying a staff, around which spirals a snake in close embrace. A later version, the Caduceus, consists of a rod about which two serpents are entwined, topped by a pair of wings. This was the magical wand of the trickster god Hermes who inhabited the liminal space between life and death and conducted souls into the afterlife. Both symbols are still used by health care organisations, though they are hardly the stuff of modern medicine.

When I first started at medical school, we new students were given a tour of the library. I liked its fustiness, its mahogany bookshelves, the desks where you could quietly study and the rows of weighty medical tomes, weighty both in size and prose. The person showing us around drew our attention to a piece of writing, modestly framed and hung up on a wall where you might not notice it if you didn't look. It was the famous Hippocratic Oath which newly qualified doctors used to take, and still do in a modified form in some countries, even though, sadly, Hippocrates was not the author. While it is still much respected for its ethical stance, if you look at what it says it has some surprises. Thus, it begins by invoking the gods Apollo, Asklepios, Hygeia and Panacea, who, I think, would make uncomfortable bedfellows with our present day clinical practice; our current medical gods might include randomised clinical trials, evidence-based medicine or vaccination, for example, but certainly not pagan deities.

I don't know how many thousands of times I have written the letters Rx. These are inscribed at the beginning of prescriptions by all doctors. Some consider it to be short for the Latin 'recipe' meaning 'to take'. Its origins, though, are in Ancient Egyptian medicine. This was brought home to me by a gift I was given as a child. It was a small piece of vivid green stone with an eye drawn in black on it. It was from Ancient Egypt and the stylised pictogram did indeed look like Rx. It represented the Eye of Horus, and was used to invoke protection from that healing god as part of prescribing treatments for a sick person. I wonder how many doctors realise this when they prescribe for their patients; the very thought of invoking an ancient, protective deity would most likely be as foreign to them as the dark side of the moon.

How is it that these mythic traces from the past still persist in modern clinical practice? One way of looking at this is to see them as Freudian slips. Freud noticed that his patients would sometimes make mistakes as they spoke; these 'errors', however, were not random. They usually gave a clue to unconscious conflicts which surfaced from time to time, rather like unpredictable, volcanic steam vents. Are they, then, signs of a repressed conflict, a dissociation in the Western medical paradigm?

I recall watching a consultant physician, later to become a professor, teaching us medical students – there were around eight of us – at the bedside of a woman with recurrent pancreatic cancer, as part of his ward round. He was young, perhaps in his forties, confident, energetic and knowledgeable. She was elderly, grey-haired, thin and quietly anxious. Her abdomen was exposed to the ward's view while he taught – for perhaps 15 or 20 minutes. The curtains were not drawn. The word cancer was never used; euphemisms such as 'mitotic lesion' or 'neoplasm' were substituted. The other patients – it was an open Nightingale ward – listened, I imagine, with much interest. He then examined her and pressed hard on her abdomen, using his weight to palpate more deeply; the diffuse nature of the tumour made it difficult to delineate. This was obviously painful for her

– I found myself wincing as I watched – and she was in pain for some hours afterwards. The consultant talked to her briefly about further investigations but didn't refer to the discussion he had led on her condition in front of her. In short, his application of medical science to her case was highly competent, but he treated her as an object, not a person. Her privacy had been invaded. Her naked abdomen was exposed to the ward (all right for some but not, perhaps, for a modest, elderly woman). She had not been asked if she had any questions about her illness. He had caused her unnecessary pain. All of this, it should be said, was done with the best of intentions. He would not have thought anything was amiss.

To me, what was missing was an empathic connection with the ill woman. How was it, I wondered, that such an academically talented research physician paid no emotional heed to his patient. Was he in some way personally lacking in such skills or was it a sign of a deficit in his medical education?

But it doesn't have to be like that. Here is a story from India. Dr Paul Brand pioneered new surgical techniques in that country to help lepers, for example by restoring function to their hands:

A few months after we opened the [leprosy] unit I was examining the hands of a bright young man, trying to explain to him in my broken Tamil that we could halt the progress of the disease, and perhaps restore some movement to his hand, but we could do little about his facial deformities. I joked a bit, laying my hand on his shoulder... I expected him to smile in response, but instead he began to shake with muffled sobs. "Have I said something wrong?" I asked my assistant in English. "Did he misunderstand me?" She quizzed him in a spurt of Tamil and reported, "No, doctor. He says he is crying because you put your hand around his shoulder. Until he came here no one had touched him for many years."
(Yancey and Brand 1997, p. 106)

Like any other doctor I've seen many horrifying sights and I had to learn to protect myself emotionally. The unspoken teaching I received was of objectivity, of standing back and observing dispassionately, of suppression of the natural human feelings that arise when in the presence of severe injuries, life-threatening illnesses, the dying, the dead. All useful of course, but they didn't help me with the nightmares I used to have about my medical experiences.

Some physicians, however, have followed a different path. William Carlos Williams (1967, p. 287) was an American poet and doctor – he worked both as a paediatrician and general practitioner. He had this to say in his autobiography:

I found by practice, by trial and error, that to treat a man as something to which surgery, drugs and hoodoo applied was an indifferent matter; to treat him as a material for a work of art made him somehow come alive to me.

A work of art, then; a melding of science and artifice. But, there's more. Let's look at the testimony of a doctor who has undergone extreme experiences. Photographs of Viktor Frankl, who was a professor of neurology and psychiatry in Vienna, show a white-haired bespectacled man, quite ordinary-looking in fact. There is no hint in them that he survived three years of internment in Auschwitz, Dachau and other concentration camps during the Second World War. One way that he stayed alive was to observe the behaviour of the inmates and guards as if he were preparing a talk to be given at a psychiatric convention. He saw that those prisoners who had some sense of meaning in their lives were more likely to survive than those who had given up hope. This was even more important than physical strength. For Frankl (2004, p. 48) himself, it was his memories of his wife that kept him going:

But my mind clung to my wife's image, imagining it with an uncanny acuteness. I heard her answering me, saw her smile, her frank and encouraging look. Real or not, her look was then more luminous than the sun which was beginning to rise.

After the war, he developed a psychological therapy called logotherapy, based on the search for meaning that is part of every person's life.

Such stories are powerful in part because they reveal something of the remarkable depths of people faced with life-threatening adversity, their courage, their tenacity and their determination.

Sigmund Freud, who looks at us out of the many photographs of him with his clever, watchful, thoughtful eyes, his clipped beard and the ever-present cigars which were to be the cause of his death from mouth cancer, thought that nine-tenths of our psyche is unconscious. Imagine, then, that you are some creature of the Antarctic, a seal perhaps, blubbered and close-furred against the freezing seas. Imagine that you are sitting at the top of a blue-white iceberg cliff a hundred feet high, that you dive down into the sea, down and down, looking for the bottom of the frozen giant. It is there, of course, but nine hundred feet down in total blackness.

There is a picture of Carl Jung (1964, p. 52) which shows him on an expedition to visit the tribesmen of Mount Elgon, Kenya in 1926. It was part of his psychological studies of traditional societies. He is wearing a solar topee, knee-length, rumpled khaki shorts and a bush shirt. In his hand he clutches his habitual pipe (which may have contributed to his later heart disease). Two white men similarly dressed stand on either side of him; six Africans, some in military uniform, and one holding a rifle, flank them. This was no package holiday; there were risks. This is an apt image, for Jung explored the unconscious with as much drive as he did the ancient cultures of the world. And he found an immense world, as varied, beautiful, ugly, dangerous, life-affirming, deadly, soulful, inspiring, puzzling and just plain strange as anything on our outer planet. Like Freud, he was at pains to point out its vastness. In a striking image, he imagined the ego with its everyday consciousness to be like a cork floating on a vast ocean representing the unconscious. We are so focused on our everyday concerns that we miss the fact that all about us is an immense, ever-changing inner seascape stretching to the horizon in every direction.

When I say he studied the unconscious, this was no mere academic exercise. In addition to his therapeutic work with his patients and their dreams, he quite literally plunged into his own unconscious. In 1913 he was troubled by a series of dreams and fantasy images which seemed to foretell the onset of the First World War. In one he saw the land between Switzerland and the North Sea flooded, the water turning to blood, with a host of drowned bodies. He felt he had to face these overpowering images. On 12 December 1913:

> I resolved upon the decisive step. I was sitting at my desk once more, thinking over my fears. Then I let myself drop. Suddenly it was as though the ground literally gave way beneath my feet, and I plunged down into dark depths. I could not fend off a feeling of panic. But then, abruptly, at not too great a depth, I landed on my feet...
> (Jung 1983, pp. 199–203)

What he found there was not a complex thinking machine but a psyche that expressed itself in myths and symbols, in stories and metaphors. And they were powerful, powerful in the way that we find a piece of music, the Blues say, causes us to shiver and feel its soulfulness, powerful in the way that we can watch old news footage of the Hiroshima atom bomb and be awed and horrified by its destructive might, powerful in the way that green fields and trees have grown again where there was once a grey-brown hell of trenches, barbed wire and shell holes among which soldiers fought during the First World War, powerful in the way that we can fall in love and be consumed by that overwhelming passion.

This unconscious psyche, then, speaks of healing through odd symbols such as a serpent wound round a staff, or creates an image and mythic story of a god to encapsulate our drive to cure. A strange language, but important, so important that it survives, even if unrecognised, every time a doctor writes Rx.

It's not that the science is unimportant. It's vital. The temptation, though, is to think that that is all there is, to split off the other aspect of our psyche and discard it. The American writer, Rebecca Solnit (2013, p. 248) comments: "Sometimes an extraordinary or huge question comes along and we try to marry it off to a mediocre answer." Telling a patient that the treatment recommended for his cancer may give him an extra four months of life, useful though that information might be, doesn't quite cut it if he's wondering what it's like to die, wondering if there is a God, wondering how he'll respond to the treatment, wondering if he'll suffer, wondering what will become of his young family.

After surgery, great care is taken to look after the vulnerable, healing body and its physiology – blood tests, ventilation, antibiotics, intravenous fluids and so on. It's the same with the psyche. It is affected by life-threatening confrontations with illness. It, too, needs a space for its care. What is required? It's simple enough: kindness and understanding and the willingness to empathise with a patient in crisis. Maybe not to have the answers to the big existential questions, but at least to listen. And patience – patients may be so shocked by the information they've been given that they forget and need to hear the same thing many times. Time, too, enough time to sit quietly and unhurriedly with a human being facing a threat to his very life. He is, after all, as William Carlos Williams said, a work of art.

But it can be painful to do that, to enter an ill person's inner world. No wonder many doctors go for the facts: armour-plating, objectivity. Still, we physicians are no less vulnerable behind the screens we put up. It would be easy to caricature that young consultant – and his lack of communication with the old woman and her cancer – as being somehow permanently defective, lacking an empathy bump in his brain, a stereotypical cartoon figure. Perhaps, though, there were other patients with whom he found he could make contact emotionally; perhaps he had suffered the gnawing anxiety that any parent feels when their child is ill; perhaps he had grieved for the loss of a loved one; perhaps many perhapses.

So, let's change the image. Let's take away all the accoutrements and pare down our picture to two human beings facing each other and facing together illness, life, death and healing. For the moment one is in the role of healer and the other the sick person. No matter. It may change soon; the healer may become ill, the patient may be healed. We could also see them as two people, each containing that immense inner seascape of the psyche that Jung wrote about. Wouldn't it be remarkable to meet at that level of truth?

Bedside Manners

Some years ago, I had to go into hospital for a minor operation. I rather liked the ward – it was large, circular and with about twenty-five beds in it. My stay gave me a taste of being on the receiving end of health care. My first encounter was with the house surgeon clerking me in. He was polite, efficient and impersonal. I didn't blame him; he was busy and had many more patients to prepare for surgery. I was just one more on the list to see. I felt, though, that we passed like two ships in the night.

The next morning, early, I donned a chilly theatre gown, the sort that leaves the whole of the back of you exposed to the world. Shortly afterwards a young student nurse came along to give me my pre-med injection. I was looking forward to this. I had been prescribing opioids (morphine-like drugs) for many years and I was anticipating finding out at first-hand what this felt like. The thought of being wheeled down to theatre in a haze of euphoria seemed an excellent one. I bared a buttock for her to administer the medication. The needle went in, but then, as she pressed the plunger, the syringe disconnected from the needle and most of my precious pre-med squirted uselessly on to the bed. The nurse was very upset and she ran off to ask the ward sister's advice. Shortly afterwards she returned, trembling, frightened and close to tears, and apologised for her mistake. My heart went out to her and I reassured her as best I could that it was not a problem. True, I was secretly disappointed at missing my first ever fix, but the ward sister had decreed that I was not to have another injection and who was I to argue with a London hospital ward sister?

Shortly afterwards I was wheeled down to the operating theatre. The anaesthetist came in, a serious, grey-haired, tough-looking woman, sniffing from a blocked nose and a cold. She looked at me as if my existence was somehow offensive to her and said: "You look even worse than I feel." With these encouraging words, she inserted an intravenous cannula into my arm. An assistant handed her the syringe filled with the induction anaesthetic. She connected this to the cannula and pushed it in fast. Unfortunately, the anaesthetic agent had only just been taken out of the fridge and was ice cold. As it shot up the veins in my forearm, it caused such intense pain that I cried out. I had no idea that there were pain receptors inside veins, but I had now discovered this to be a fact. As the anaesthetic began to take effect, I had a strange image of inhabiting a dark space through which grey clouds were rolling – as though this were the anaesthetic flowing through my brain. I then lost consciousness.

I was awakened by pain – a theatre nurse was pulling off the electrode monitoring my heart from the skin of my chest. I was as helpless as a baby and when they lifted me on to the gurney, I couldn't move my limbs, they were so relaxed from the anaesthetic. As they pushed the gurney back, I had the sensation that I had somehow dived below heavy grey clouds into a place of light and felt wonderfully comfortable. Afterwards, the surgeon came to my bed where I was sleeping off the drugs and told me that the operation had gone well. I so appreciated him doing this.

I suppose this is not out of the ordinary as hospital experiences go – and, after all, the operation was a success. But to me it highlighted the difference between impersonal and personal care. I felt grateful for the genuine human contact I received, but felt a mixture of amazement, anger and a sort of wry amusement at my medical colleague's thoughtlessness. The veins in my forearm had completely thrombosed and it took most of a year for some of them to heal and recanalise. It could so easily have been avoided.

That, I think, was what I have really valued about hospice work. It gives space to treat patients as people, to respond to their needs, be they medical or otherwise. These were people who had sometimes been through several taxing major operations as well as chemotherapy and radiotherapy. Their bodies had been brutally assaulted – even if for good reason. They needed care, compassionate care; they needed to be valued and respected as individuals.

While I never did get my pre-med, I did experience something rather more interesting as I was being anaesthetised. Was it really possible that my consciousness could watch the influx of anaesthetic, rolling through my awareness until I knew no more? Well, why not? My guess is that such experiences may be common. It's just that no one asks.

Some while ago, I had an MRI scan, a procedure that uses a powerful magnetic field instead of X-rays to delineate the tissues of the body. One of the radiographers came to fetch me from the waiting room. She smiled, introduced herself by name and shook my hand. She carefully checked through her list of contraindications to having a scan. All was well. I was to change into a theatre gown. We cunningly got round the problem of rear exposure: "Wear two," she said, "one front to back and the other back to front." Such genius. I felt like an extra in one of those biblical films.

Another radiographer inserted a cannula to give contrast dye during the scan. We chatted for a short while about his work. He said the injection might feel a little cold – it didn't. Lying in the scanner tunnel, I was given a panic button, and a pair of headphones to reduce the noisy vibrating, clunking and juddering as the machine went through its scanning procedure. The scan didn't trouble me though I can understand why some people feel panicky when they are in the scanner tunnel.

To me this was such a different experience. I was treated thoughtfully and with respect. My contact with the radiographers felt human and real, even though they were busy. It didn't take much; just simple courtesy.

A Perfect Baby?

We struggled to keep up with the multiple medical complications which visited this tiny baby – extreme prematurity (she was born at about 28 week gestation), respiratory infections, septicaemia, brain haemorrhages and bowel inflammation. Every time we had dealt with one crisis in our Special Care Baby Unit, another loomed. She needed high levels of oxygen through a ventilator to maintain her blood oxygenation. At one stage, there was a question of an operation for her bowels. I remember the anaesthetist coming to visit the baby and assess her fitness for operation. I remember her intent, single-minded face, her short dark hair with a quiff, her determined stance as she examined the baby, her arms plunged into the portholes that allowed access to the brilliantly lit incubator. Her irritation was apparent when she spoke. Surgery *was* possible, but she also had very decided views about the wisdom of operating on such an ill premature baby. She felt this tiny infant shouldn't have surgery – a view which had much to recommend it given how frail the baby was. She then continued: "I mean, if she survives, she'll be brain-damaged and a terrible burden to the parents. It's much better to let her go and they can have another child, who'll be a perfect baby."

There was a note of callousness in what she said, as if babies were a sort of generic model that could be discarded if imperfect like Sindy dolls. There was no sense of her being aware of what the parents wanted. She had written their child off as damaged goods and didn't seem to see this baby as a living being with her own rights. I was quietly incensed.

In the end, an operation wasn't needed. The baby had another brain haemorrhage and died shortly afterwards with her parents sitting beside her. They were deeply saddened after their long vigil by their daughter's incubator and I was relieved that they didn't have to take the agonising decision about whether their daughter should have an operation or not.

There is, however, another way of seeing this anaesthetist's intervention. I wonder if she actually found it unbearable to watch the suffering of this tiny child and her parents. I wonder whether she had developed a carapace, a sort of psychological armouring, as protection against her own pain in the face of the repeated stories of distress that she witnessed daily as a doctor. Perhaps this had contributed to her response.

The Fall of Icarus

I was once asked to visit a patient dying of cancer because he wouldn't stop talking. This was a unique referral and in hindsight I would have done better to listen to my uneasiness, the subtle feeling that something wasn't quite right. Instead I imagined it just meant he had a lot to say about his illness. As I climbed the narrow stairs of his house I could hear his voice, a continual rising and falling cadence. When I walked into his bedroom, I found his mother sitting in a chair beside his bed quietly listening. His body was wasted and his face gaunt. I gathered he hadn't stopped for several days and his family took it in turns to sit with him – he was calmer that way. He did not pause while I was introduced to him. I asked to sit with him. It was obvious to me that he displayed the typical signs of mania. He would go off along one train of thought, and then another notion came to him and he branched off into that idea. This endlessly repeated sequence is called flight of ideas in medical parlance. What he talked about was very elevated – he seemed to be trying to discover the meaning of his life – but he wasn't able to hold the thread of his reflections together. When I tried to intervene, and have a dialogue with him, he became highly irritated, another feature of mania. His words now became more and more tinged with anger. He had been an amateur boxer when he was younger, he told me, and he threatened to go several rounds with me. Now, I am no boxer, but he was emaciated and dying so I felt reasonably confident I could stave off an attack. His grasp of reality was tenuous – he seemed to have no sense that his behaviour was abnormal. There was a sense of the grandiose in what he said, again a feature of mania. He became increasingly agitated, and I retreated down the stairs followed by him punching the woodwork.

I could see he was about to attack me and I was compelled to restrain him. He got in a punch which made my head sing – he had a surprising amount of strength despite his frail condition. As soon as he was on the ground, astonishingly he began whimpering like a little child and begging me not to hurt him. It was as though the wings that bore up his manic flight had fallen from him and he fell, like Icarus, into the sea of reality. He had to be temporarily admitted to a psychiatric unit where he was treated with antipsychotic medication which calmed him but did not halt his endless conversations, often with himself. My abiding memory is of seeing him sitting in bed in a single room in the hospice, alone and quietly muttering to himself. I feel sad as I remember him. While his distress was reduced, I wish there had been some way of reaching him on a human level, even in the midst of the overwhelming torrent of his tumbling thoughts.

What brought about this dramatic behaviour? It would be easy to dismiss this with a psychiatric diagnosis: manic psychosis. But this is just a description, saying in effect that his psyche was racing and he had lost contact with everyday reality. What was also striking was his attempts to find some meaning in his plight. It was as though he were trying to steer a car down a steep hill with the accelerator pedal stuck at full on and no brakes. I wondered if his confrontation with his mortal illness had plunged him into an existential crisis such that his ego could not cope with the powerful, unconscious forces that were surging through him.

In hindsight I think his mother understood best. She just sat and listened.

Diogenes

Many religious traditions talk about non-attachment as an inner attitude that brings freedom. Most of us, however, struggle along with our attachments.

One family I encountered, however, took attachment to its limits. When I was working as a junior doctor in geriatrics, my consultant took me out on a domiciliary visit. He didn't tell me anything beforehand – I think, in retrospect, this was a bit of showmanship. The house, when we came to it, was very ordinary – 1930s terraced – with scaffolding up and repair work going on. It was when we went inside that I saw why we had come. Every inch of the hall, the combined sitting and living room and kitchen was covered with the detritus of years. There were towering columns of magazines and yellowing newspapers, books, cardboard boxes of varied ages and prove-nances, clothes, ornaments, furniture, bits of furniture, kitchen implements, parts of kitchen implements, crockery, cutlery, nuts and bolts, indeterminate bits of machinery, most covered in years of dust. And, in the midst of this sea of rubbish, stood, like jewels glittering in a sty, a gleaming new white washing machine and an equally shiny fridge.

The elderly man who had let us in – a very ordinary-looking person whom I would never have suspected of being a serial hoarder – then led us upstairs to see his sister, whose illness had led her general practitioner to request this domiciliary visit. As we negotiated the stairs and the landing, we squeezed between more dusty piles of the fossilised past. We entered her bedroom. She lay in bed, frail and small, her long, grey hair flowing down the pillows. To my astonishment I saw that, around the walls of the bedroom, a thick rampart about three feet high had been constructed, mostly of dingy clothes, but supported by further newspapers. There was a musty smell in the air. I looked at her sheets and pillows. They were brown. Then I looked again. I saw they had actually once been white and now, after I don't know how many months or years of uninterrupted use, had become dark, 'engrimed' by constant human contact.

She looked to me, for reasons I can't quite ascertain, like a lost princess, old, sad and alone, locked away in the dungeon of her and her brother's desperate, if unconscious, clinging to anything and everything that spelled security and safety, that made them forget their atavistic fear of, what? Poverty, destitution, hunger, sickness? They probably didn't know themselves. They were a kind of modern Hansel and Gretel. Despite their squalor, my heart went out to her. I can't remember what her physical illness was, but maybe that was less important than her extraordinary situation. My consultant, crisp and clinical, told me afterwards this was a case of the Diogenes syndrome, named after a Greek philosopher who lived, with his few possessions, in a barrel. It didn't seem a very apt name to me. Diogenes was trying to lead the simple life with as few belongings as possible; though, no doubt, it would still have been cramped in his chosen residence.

Her story makes me think, rather guiltily, of all those possessions I have kept 'just in case', a sort of Second World War mentality when even used bits of string and paper used to be kept.

There is a story from the East about a thief who broke into the dwelling of a holy man. On the table was a bowl filled with precious stones – diamonds, sapphires and rubies. "Please," said the holy man, waving his arm expansively, "help yourself. Take whatever you wish." The thief needed no prompting and seized the bowl, poured the jewels into his pocket and ran off, congratulating himself on his good fortune. About a week later there was a knock at the holy man's door. He opened it. The thief stood outside, his head bowed. "What!" said the holy man. "You want more? I haven't got anything left to give you." The thief replied, shame-faced: "I want whatever it is that gives you the freedom to let go of those jewels."

The Snack Break

Patients' behaviour can seem like an incomprehensible cipher at times. Take Richard for example. He had been admitted for surgery to the ward where I was working as a newly qualified house surgeon. All went well at first. I clerked him in and the next day he went down to the operating theatre for surgery. It was during the days following that things started to go wrong. The nurses reported his increasingly erratic behaviour and his picking at his stitches so that they came undone and the good work carried out surgically was nullified. One night, my wife was the duty surgical officer and she was called to the ward. Richard was unwell and required an X-ray. He was also even more uncooperative than usual. My wife felt she and a porter should accompany him to the X-ray Department because of this. As they walked down the ward, he suddenly turned right, reached for the thermometer beside a patient's bed and swallowed it. My wife shepherded him back to the central aisle of the ward but he made a break left and helped himself to another thermometer. The nurses were now deploying at speed to keep him away from the other ward thermometers. Sometimes they succeeded, sometimes he was too quick for them. At last they got him out of the ward, but Richard wasn't finished yet. There was a window with a broken pane of glass. He reached out, broke off several shards and ate them as well.

The next day he was calmer, having received a hefty dose of antipsychotic medication.

It was not possible to talk with him about this incident. He was psychotic and had no insight into his behaviour. We did, however, send him for an X-ray and saw the various bits of glass and blobs of mercury situated in different parts of his intestines. We were concerned that the glass would perforate his bowel but it never did. Neither did he develop symptoms of mercury poisoning, though this was hard to assess because of his psychosis. We took serial X-rays and watched the progress of his vitreous snack with fascination. Even passing them in his bowel motions didn't cause any damage. I was astonished at the resilience of his guts.

We never discovered the origins of this extraordinary self-harming behaviour. It seems likely that such terrible violence directed towards himself must have been caused by a severely disturbed and abusive childhood. Painters such as Michelangelo in his *Last Judgement*, and Hieronymus Bosch in his painting called, simply, *Hell*, showed demons inflicting unspeakable tortures on their victims. The odd thing is that, as with Richard, right now around the world humans are carrying out just such unspeakable acts on each other: torture, murder, genocide, rape and child abuse. It seems it isn't necessary to wait for the Last Judgement. The tentacles of Hell are only a news flash away.

Perhaps that is why I became a doctor – healing rather than hell.

Chapter 5

Suffering

When I look to discovering a meaning in suffering, I find myself turning to the sick people I have worked with. I see an endless line of individuals moving through the landscape of my mind:

Soon after she is born, it becomes obvious that she can't swallow. Investigations show a congenital blockage of her oesophagus which needs immediate surgery. I come down to the recovery room to take her back to the Special Care Baby Unit after surgery. She is pale blue and floppy, and despite maximum ventilation her blood oxygen levels are critically low. The anaesthetist has run out of options. Feeling we have nothing to lose, I change the ventilation tube. At once she starts to pink up. The previous tube was blocked by clotted blood. I feel a shiver of excitement: she is going to make it, I think, and she does.

He is six foot, four inches tall. His once powerful physique has melted away to skin and bones. He is confused and wandering aimlessly around the ward. I take him by the hand and lead him back to his bed. I can feel the residue of his strength in his grip. I'm relieved that he isn't resisting. Before he became ill he could have thrown me across the room.

She is eight years old and has Down's syndrome. She has been admitted with a congenital cardiac disorder and a respiratory infection. When her breathing is comfortable she is a delight, sociable, playful and talkative. When she gets short of breath, she gets crotchety. She goes a pale, greyish-blue colour; she has to sit upright in bed to ease her distress. She doesn't move; her breathing won't allow it.

And so the queue continues... What can we say? Their suffering happened; they didn't want it but they lived with it and accepted what was inevitable. Their courage and dignity moved me. I felt they were, without knowing it, teaching us how to live.

Many animals care for their young, but we do more. We care for our sick, wounded and dying. This isn't a calculated response. It's instinctive, a response born of compassion.

Fabiola was a rich and beautiful Roman noblewoman who lived in the 4th century AD. She was a Christian convert and used her wealth to build the first hospital and the first hospice in the West. But this was not charity at a distance. St Jerome (1933, p. 323) gives this description of her:

> She founded an infirmary and gathered into it sufferers from the streets, giving their poor bodies worn with sickness and hunger all a nurse's care. How often did she carry on her own shoulders poor filthy wretches tortured by epilepsy! How often did she wash away the purulent matter from wounds which others could not even endure to look upon! She gave food from her own hand, and even when a man was but a breathing corpse, she would moisten his lips with drops of water.

Even in extreme circumstances this can hold good. Father Maximilian Kolbe, a Polish Catholic priest, was imprisoned in Auschwitz for hiding Jews during the Second World War. Following the disappearance of three prisoners, the deputy camp commandant, thinking they had escaped, chose ten prisoners to be locked in the Bunker, an underground cell in Block 13 and starved to death as a deterrent. One of the men chosen broke down, lamenting the loss of his wife and children. Father Maximilian stepped forward and offered himself as a substitute.

Remarkably, the commandant accepted. In the starvation cell, Father Maximilian supported the other prisoners: sounds of singing and prayer were heard coming out of the cell. After two weeks he was the only one left alive and was murdered by lethal injection. The man whose life he saved lived on until 1995; he was 95 years old when he died.

Sometimes suffering is radically transformed. Eckhart Tolle (1999, pp. 1–2) gives a vivid description of this:

Until my thirtieth year, I lived in a state of almost continuous anxiety interspersed with periods of suicidal depression... One night, I woke up in the early hours with a feeling of absolute dread... "I cannot live with myself any longer." This was the thought that kept repeating itself... Then suddenly I became aware of what a peculiar thought it was. "Am I one or two? If I cannot live with myself, there must be two of me: the 'I' and the 'self' that 'I' cannot live with." "Maybe," I thought, "only one of them is real." I was so stunned by this strange realisation that my mind stopped... I felt drawn in to what seemed a vortex of energy... Suddenly there was no more fear, and I let myself fall into the void. I was awakened by the chirping of a bird... The first light was filtering through the curtain... That soft luminosity was love itself. Tears came into my eyes... Everything was fresh and pristine as if it had just come into existence. That day I walked around the city in utter amazement at the miracle of life on earth.

Listen Up

Yes, listen. In childhood, this isn't just a useful skill; it is vital for a child's development. A child psychotherapist called Virginia Axline (1971) anatomised this necessity in a moving book called *Dibs*.

It tells the story of Dibs a disturbed six year old child who was thought to be either mentally retarded, brain-damaged or autistic. In therapy, it became apparent that he was in fact an intellectually gifted, sensitive and creative child. A psychiatrist told his parents he was not retarded, but "the most rejected and emotionally deprived child he had ever seen" (p. 76). Dibs' parents didn't agree.

Axline used play therapy with Dibs. She sat quietly and listened, mirroring back to him what he said or did. She used a sand tray: Dibs was invited to play with model humans or animals of his choosing placed in the sand. As he moved them around, he acted out the stories he found so difficult to tell in words. Or he would paint, perhaps talking about the images he produced and she would let him know he had her full attention by reflecting back to him his words. He came to know that another human being had heard him, that he existed. In these ways the stories of his life and the traumas he had experienced came to light. Under the warm sun of her unwavering attention he healed and flourished, and a very different child emerged: intelligent, thoughtful, creative and loving.

Some while after Dibs' psychotherapy had been completed, Virginia Axline met him by chance in the street. They reminisced about the work they had done together. She asked him:

"'What did we play, Dibs?' Dibs leaned towards me. His eyes were shining. 'Everything I did, you did,' he whispered. 'Everything I said, you said.'" (p. 190)

He had come to know himself through her, and to know that

he was loved – and lovable.

Listening needs commitment. No half measures here, no eyes sliding off to look at the newspaper on a nearby chair, no inner fantasy to distract you. No, listening isn't like that. It's active – even if you're silent. There she is, your patient or client or friend, sitting before you talking. you're taking in her every word, intently, with all the understanding you can muster, entering her world, whether it is deadly or sane, large or luxurious, sad or hilarious; there's no end to the possibilities. And as you listen, you become at one with her. She becomes human, real, no matter what her story – and boy do people have stories, long ones and short ones, sad ones to make you cry or so funny you'd want to laugh till your sides ache, haunting ones that make you go cold and shiver with fear and beautiful ones that make you sigh with pleasure; every variety under the sun – which has seen it all.

It's what we do, it's about our memories, what happened to us, or rather what we perceive happened to us, upon which our emotions depend. "And then he died," she says and weeps silent, bitter tears. "And then, God knows how, she pulled through," he says and his relief is almost palpable and his lately frozen face melts and relaxes.

And we have to tell someone. We must speak our pent-up tale or, what? Or die? Well, no, but instead that feeling of loneliness, that yawning, dark, inner space that is akin to death. We are a social species, we must talk, we must know that another listens, sympathises, gives of their time willingly and lovingly.

Even in the womb where for soul aeons we floated weightless and timeless, we heard our mother's heartbeat – such a steady and reassuring speech – and the distant murmur of sounds from the unknown world and the dim, rust light that filters through the thin barrier of flesh between us and the future. We are in connection; all is well.

And so we are born and held and soothed while our voice – our babbling, laughing, crying, roaring even – is heard and our parents mirror this back to us, solicitous, empathising, grimacing in sympathy when we are in pain, laughing when we laugh, repeating back to us our sounds and half-words – those unconscious vowels and syllables – as we la-la-la to them and to the vast world into which we have been born.

Yes, we need to be listened to, or we die inside. Untended, children sicken and fade away. We need each other. Why, the very development of a child's brain depends on this loving and crucial connection, interaction, love, intercourse, togetherness. All of that.

Lifelong, it doesn't change. And we take our turn too, what we have been taught we do; we know a friend is in trouble, we listen, empathise, are silent, suggest, smile, share in the sadness. Yes, that.

And when you're old and ill, especially if you're ill, you need this. You don't care about medical insights into the physics of sound vibrations sine-waving through the invisible air to be received by the shell of an ear and translated into meaning in the infinite interstices of our extraordinary brain. No, you are hurt, lonely, melancholic, frightened. What you care about is when the numberless bits of sound are transformed into: "Yes," said so gently, or "I understand." Well, thank God someone does.

Who's Who?

We tend to think that roles in medicine are clearly demarcated. The patient is ill and needs curing. The doctor is well and does the curing. End of story. Or is it?

I was on a ward round as a junior doctor following my consultant and senior registrar around an echoing Nightingale ward, accompanied by a group of medical students and watched apprehensively by the other patients, who were sitting by or lying in their beds depending on how sick they were, waiting for their turn to be seen. We came to the bed of a man of about forty, dark-haired, well-looking. He had a testicular cancer. He was a courageous and thoughtful man and had already insisted in knowing what was wrong with him, something that not many patients did at that time. Now he wanted to know what treatment was available and what his chances were. The consultant, usually supremely confident and a highly experienced teacher, was reduced to a state of inarticulate stuttering. I had never seen him like this. Eventually he said that no one is a statistic, by which I think he meant that whatever the odds, there is a chance of survival. We moved on leaving the patient to muse on this fragment of information. Later, we all sat in the ward sister's office drinking a cup of coffee – part of the ward round ritual. The consultant had regained some of his ebullience and, setting down his coffee cup, said: "He won't do well. Patients have got to have faith in their doctors. He won't do well." Even I, an inexperienced junior doctor, could recognise the attempt, albeit unconscious, to blame the patient for asking too many questions. I didn't think the patient lacked faith; he just wanted to know how best to treat his illness and to make provision for the future.

At face value, this sounds like an embarrassing exercise in medical non-communication or perhaps anti-communication.

However, I knew that this same consultant had been diagnosed with a malignancy some months before and had been away on sick leave while he had chemotherapy and convalesced. I realised that when he was questioned so closely by the patient, his distress at his own illness surfaced, rendering him unable to speak for a little. When he said that no one is a statistic, these were, I think, his own words for his own comfort. Suddenly, he was in the role of the patient. He had been sick and struggled with his own fears of dying. He had looked for hope. And he had, probably unwittingly, passed on his own mantra to his interlocutor.

So, who is the patient? Who is the healer? I think we all are both at different times. The names actually cover a much wider conceptualisation of sickness and healing than that of traditional medical practice. We become ill in protean ways, many of which cannot be comfortably assigned to a diagnostic box in a medical textbook. Healing, too, is not bounded by a medical qualification. Apart from the plethora of therapies now on offer – such as psychotherapy, physiotherapy, nutrition, massage, aromatherapy and acupuncture – this is something we do for each other every day, very simply, often without even realising: listening, a hug, a massage, companionship, walking together, a mutual insight into some difficult problem, humour, a shared 'aha' moment.

Doctors get ill like everyone else. This is still seen as a stigma, which is a pity because, like nothing else, sickness teaches you what it is like to live with a particular diagnosis, whether this be heart disease, cancer, depression or rheumatoid arthritis. I would far rather be treated for an illness by a doctor who has gone through the same illness herself or, in fact, who has gone through *any* significant illness. I would so value the shared experience – vital in providing compassionate as well as scientific care. A wounded healer brings an irreplaceable dimension to care of the sick.

The Operation

I still feel anger when I remember the story of this little girl, even though it was over 30 years ago. She weighed a little over 800 grams at birth when she was admitted to the Special Care Baby Unit in which I was working, and this dropped to about 750 grams later. Just a hand full. She was very premature: about 27 weeks' gestation, instead of the usual 40 weeks. I remember particularly that she was a very active baby despite being so premature; she would wave her limbs and move her head more than other babies on the unit. With the medical technology available at that time, her chances of survival were low. And she did indeed have what doctors euphemistically call a stormy time; in other words, she nearly died. Myself and the other junior doctor working with me on the unit were fully occupied keeping her intravenous infusions going in her tiny veins – putting a drip up on her was the reverse of threading a needle, it was like trying to get a needle into a thread – and her ventilator working. She became sicker and sicker. Her respiratory function was badly compromised and she had life-threatening infections. And then another crisis struck. She developed necrotising enterocolitis, a dreaded and potentially lethal condition where parts of the bowel die. Surgery may be needed to remove the dead bowel. In a tiny premature baby, this is obviously a major undertaking. Despite our more conservative endeavours, she deteriorated and surgery became necessary.

When she came back from surgery, she was obviously intensely agitated and moving her limbs even more, and one of the nurses remarked that her pulse rate was 250 beats a minute. (The normal resting rate in adults is 70 beats a minute. Newborn babies might run at 120 to 160 beats per minute.) As we tried to work out the cause of this, the reason became clear. Prior to her operation she had received a drug to paralyse her, but not any anaesthetic. It was no wonder her pulse was so high. She had gone through the operation with nothing to prevent her feeling pain. I remember feeling a mixture of disbelief, anger and a sorrow that she had had to go through such an experience. I learned later that this was common practice in anaesthetics then. The medical view was that very premature babies didn't feel much pain, didn't remember it and also that they didn't tolerate anaesthetics well. Ask any mother of a premature baby if he feels pain. She would look at you as if you had taken leave of your senses. Of course he feels pain, she might say; look how he cried when you took that blood sample or set up that drip.

This was one occasion when, as a junior doctor who was not supposed to, I felt so impassioned that I spoke out. I could feel the sense of hesitation among the rest of the team. This was always how it had been done. Anaesthetists had written papers on the risks of anaesthetics for premature babies. Long discussions followed. In the end the policy did change.

In 1963, Stanley Milgram, a Yale University psychologist, set up a controversial experiment in which study subjects, who were told they were taking part in a memory experiment, administered graded electric shocks to 'learners' when they got answers wrong. These 'learners' were in fact actors who were not actually receiving shocks. The subjects heard sounds of distress as the voltage of the 'shock' increased. The remarkable thing was that they kept administering higher and higher levels of electric shocks in obedience to the experimenter, even though they thought they were causing severe pain. (Milgram 1974)

While this study was clearly unethical, it does show we tend to obey authority figures even against our own judgement and conscience. Perhaps this goes some way to explaining how it could come about that babies were not given anaesthetics during operations. Received medical wisdom in the shape of authoritative textbooks and established practice says it is like this; therefore it must be like this. It doesn't matter if a baby is distressed and crying in pain, their carers think, those are only grimaces such as all babies make. It is an example of preconceptions distorting perception of reality and of a catastrophic denial of empathy. Buddhists talk about Beginner's Mind to describe someone who sees things just as they are. In the story of the Emperor's new clothes, it is a child, with his Beginner's Mind, who sees the truth. Babies know when they are hurting; we need only listen to them.

Her pulse did slow down and she did survive. She remained a wriggler which, it seemed to me, meant she was a fighter: all to the good for her future, then. I sometimes wonder what happened to her. She survived thanks to the highly skilled medical and surgical interventions she received, but what aftereffects was she left with following her dramatic entry into life?

Ancestors' Voices

When Amelia was brought into the palliative care unit, it was obvious that her older sister, Winnie, had cared for her devotedly over the nine months during which Amelia's cancer advanced relentlessly. Her nightgown was crisp, white and ironed, and she had a small case with all her requirements packed neatly inside.

But the increasing burden of care had taken its toll on Winnie, and she had at last agreed to Amelia coming in to give her sister a break. Winnie was a serious, watchful woman originally from the British Virgin Islands, as was Amelia. Her devotion to her younger sister was obvious.

Things did not go well for Amelia. Her cancer had caught up with her. She deteriorated rapidly and died within a week of admission. To say that Winnie was heartbroken was an understatement. I have rarely seen such anguish and rage in a person. She shouted repeatedly that we had butchered her sister and refused all attempts to support her. She left the ward simmering with anger at her loss.

A little while later, her general practitioner asked if staff from the hospice would meet with Winnie to talk over what had happened. One of the nurses and I went to meet her at the general practitioner's surgery. Winifred sat in the room, separating herself from us. Her face was contorted by the violence of her feelings. She was invited by her doctor to speak about how she felt. Quiet at first, she muttered that we had butchered her sister. When we tried to enter a dialogue, her voice rose and rose till she was screaming over and over again the same words: "You have butchered her," while tears poured down her face. The experience was so extraordinarily intense that I found myself beginning to see images of blood-stained butchers' knives. Eventually she was so overwrought that she had to be taken to another room to calm down. We were deeply shaken by her raw anger.

While what Winnie said bore no resemblance to the reality of what had happened to her sister, I was left wondering how such an intensity of feeling had come about. It was the kind of thing that someone who had been deeply traumatised would say. However, I knew nothing of Winnie's earlier life, so this remained a conjecture. Perhaps, too, Amelia had been holding on to life because her sister did not want to let her go. This is a repeating theme in palliative care: the attachment and love of a family may sometimes, as it were, hold a person in life. It is when they are ready to let go that the patient, too, can let go. Admission to a palliative care unit may act as a rite of passage, facilitating such a transition.

Maybe, though, there is another level to this story. It was so extreme and overwhelming that I wondered if this was not just from Winnie alone but from what Carl Jung called the collective unconscious. In other words that her experience of loss tapped into a deeper archetypal anguish, that of the enslavement and brutalisation of her race. Such words as "butchery" then begin to make sense. Most of Amelia's carers were, in fact, white. Just as Winnie cared so solicitously for her younger sister, so did thousands upon thousands of her race, enslaved black women, who tried every way they knew how to care for and protect their families in the face of the grim realities of life on sugar and cotton plantations. Consciousness of such suffering would be more than one person could bear; it would be no wonder, then, that Winifred was taken over by her feelings. The voices of her traumatised ancestors may have been pouring through her.

Hairless

If you think about it, human hair is the most extraordinary thing. Left to grow, straight hair will reach below your buttocks. I can't think of any other animal that has hair over half its body length. You would have thought that, in hunter-gatherer times, it would have been a survival risk – getting caught in thorn bushes if you are fleeing from a predator, for example. Perhaps its advantages in sexual, grooming and social status terms made up for this.

Some years ago I decided, since a significant number of my hair follicles had gone on permanent leave, that there was nothing for it but to have a Number One. Accordingly, I made my way to New Century Gents Hairdressers. Est. 1906. Nowadays there is also a sign informing passers-by that "We've been cutting it for a century." In the windows were assorted photos of famous and not famous satisfied customers ensconced in a cape and smiling happily as their hair was cut, and a nostalgic black and white photo of the shop taken in the 1950s. Above the door they had not one, but two barbers' poles. One was lit from inside and twirled slowly. They meant business.

Men's hairdressers' shops have a particular atmosphere to them, which this one shared. I sat down on one of the chairs for those waiting and looked around. There was a pin-up on the wall of a beautiful woman – Australian – with long blond hair wearing a G-string and nothing else, staring out over a computer-generated sea in which could be seen a large shark fin impossibly close to the shore. (Freud would have had a field day with that one.) On a small table were old magazines and today's newspapers. A prominent sign said: "Clean hair is healthy hair. Have a shampoo." Another showed a poster from the 1950s, an advert for Brylcreem. A man was combing back his glossy black hair, while nearby another part of the picture showed a football player with equally glossy black hair, kneeling behind a football. One of the windows was inhabited by four potted plants, two of which were climbers and had grown to form a leafy arch. The hairdressers were working at their chrome and faux-leather chairs with complicated pumping pedals. The mirrors were crowded with family pictures and photos of customers. There was a faint, slightly musty smell of damp hair, shampoo and hair gel. On the floor were the sacrificial remains of the last customer's hair. Scissors and combs soaked in fungicidal solution, and hair products gathered dust in cabinets.

When my turn came, I sat down in my barbers' chair and asked for my Number One. On one side was a man having Just A Trim, and on the other a boy sitting on a booster chair making a face as his hair was cut while his mother watched anxiously behind him. With a flourish, my barber placed a cape around me and produced an electric razor set to Number One. As he sheared me, he asked if I had enjoyed the Arsenal match. I'm not much good at hairdresser conversations, and, shamefaced, I had to tell him that I hadn't watched it; I felt as though I had committed a major sin. (My Inner Critic came on line: "What! You should have watched!") What was I doing for the weekend? As it happened, not a lot. (Inner Critic: "Lazy!") Did I have any holidays planned? At the time I didn't. (Inner Critic: "Disorganised!") Having exhausted his introductory conversational gambits, my barber lapsed into a buzzing silence, and I gratefully joined him. With the air of a gardener determinedly dealing with rampant weeds, he attacked my eyebrow, nose and ear hair. Soon I was done and I nervously surveyed my one millimetre length hair. My head felt cool as I walked down the street.

The reactions I had to my haircut were interesting. There were no compromise views; either people liked it or they didn't. My brother was genuinely shocked and kindly told me that I was even uglier than before. What surprised me, though, was that some people who knew me quite well didn't recognise me and I got used to telling those with blank faces who I was to save further embarrassment. I had no idea that hair played such an important part in how we identify each other. It did, however, give me a slight inkling of what it felt like to lose your hair suddenly through chemotherapy.

Hair loss is such a frequent part of cancer treatment that we are all familiar with the sight on television of bald children or adults, and we know that most likely they are having chemotherapy. We know that it will grow back again, so that seems all right. But is it?

If men lose their hair naturally, it is very slow, over many years. And yet think of the expedients the male population thinks up to stave off follicular Armageddon: comb-overs, wigs, hair implants, potions. Or Grecian 2000 for those pesky greys. I recall one man who came into hospital for an operation sporting an ill-fitting wig to which he was, so to speak, very attached. On the ward round, the consultant asked him a question. The man was lying back against the pillows. He shook his head in reply. I was fascinated to see that the wig, because of its contact with the pillow, remained stationary while his head rotated. He even wore his wig during his operation.

With chemotherapy, it is nothing like this. Over the days and weeks, first a few hairs are noticed on the brush, then hair starts coming out in clumps so that the chemotherapee looks piebald, and then complete baldness.

This is particularly hard for women. You have only to glance at the multimillion pound industry around hair to realise just how valued it is. The cut: perm, bob, pageboy, spiky, punk, cane-row, dreadlocks, afro. The colour: streaked, raven, chestnut, honey blond, bleached. Think of the thousands of hairdressing salons, beauty counters in department stores and hair product sections in chemists, not to mention the adverts.

And suddenly it's all gone. Just a bald head. Oh, and quite

likely a hairless body as well.

So, what do you do? Tough it out? Defiantly walk around naked headed, as it were. Some women do, but it's hard. So maybe try covering it up – a scarf, turban, bobble hat or wig. It's still pretty obvious. Some women try wearing no head cover in private and, say, a scarf in public. Then, there's the question of how long your regrowing hair needs to be before you feel you can go out in public again.

Behind this is loss. It's encouraging that the hair will grow back again, but it is still a loss – a loss of who you thought you were, of control, of beauty, sexuality and status. You are branded, against your will, as someone with that taboo disease, cancer. People you know may cross the street to avoid you or say inappropriate things because they are so nervous they don't know what to say. Suddenly you have had a brush with mortality and you are never the same afterwards.

Of course, most women do find their way through their time of hair loss successfully and there is that moment of happiness when the first signs of hair appear again, or that time, later on, when they have grown so much hair again that they need it cut; such a sign of the body reasserting itself, of life returning.

Tyger, Tyger

On a visit to London Zoo, I was looking into the tiger enclosure. It was large, grassy, with a pool and a fallen tree trunk to climb on. Quite the thing, you would have thought, for a large carnivore. At one point there was a thick glass wall through which you could look directly into the enclosure. A tiger was padding to and fro on the other side of the transparent wall. I was standing two feet away from this huge predator with only an invisible barrier between us. I could feel my skin crawl. The tiger, however, didn't take much notice of the human spectators gawking at it. It followed a pathway perhaps fifty feet in length, parallel with the glass wall. It would hurry to one end, turn round and then hurry back to the other end. Its movements had a stereotyped quality to them which reminded me of disturbed children who rock for hours without cease. Its eyes were fixed and glazed. Its coat was matted and thick, not at all like the beautiful gold and black-striped coats of its kin in the rainforests of India. Its swift trot was nothing like the leisurely movements of wild tigers in their natural environment.

Tigers range hundreds of miles in their forest habitat. This tiger's instinctive drive to do just that had been frustrated, leaving only an atavistic urge to move, however restricted the surroundings. If it had been human, I would have said it was showing traumatic behaviour.

I liked Gwyneth very much. She was a tall, thin 70 year old woman, quite shy, but kindly and gentle too. She reminded me of a deer. The first warning I had of trouble was when she told me, her general practitioner, about frequent and vivid dreams. These were soon followed by hallucinations at night which kept her awake. A sedative helped to keep these symptoms at bay for a while. Over the next weeks and months she became more and more forgetful and it became clear that she was developing dementia. Eventually she had to be admitted to a long-stay ward because she could no longer cope independently. As the months went by she found it increasingly difficult to rest and would spend most of her time walking up and down the ward. She even left the ward at times. Once she was found a mile or two away walking along a busy main road. It was as if she were on her own inner migration, like the doe-eyed caribou, the migratory deer of Arctic Canada which journey thousands of miles each year. The exit to the ward had to be barred for her safety.

She became even thinner as a result of her constant pacing. Her eyes had a fixed look to them as if she were in search of something which she had lost. Eventually tranquillisers were needed to reduce her automaton-like marching behaviour and to allow her to rest. It was the least bad alternative.

It seems to me that she and the tiger had this in common: they were both caged, she by her failing mind and it by its enclosure. There was the same pacing, the same fixed look, the same urgency. Maybe the famous lines written by William Blake (1970, p. 101) are as much about the human need for liberty as they are about the wildness of an animal.

Tyger, tyger, burning bright,
In the forests of the night...

Blake's poem was about a hunter but deer, too, which Gwyneth so much resembled, are wild creatures and have just as much need for freedom as tigers.

The Scream

Night had fallen on the medical ward where I was working. I say medical; actually it was part of an old TB hospital which had two-storey wards built like ribs off an invisible central spine and with balconies at the end where TB patients could take the air to help their recovery. A patient, an African man with a heart condition, unexpectedly had a cardiac arrest and died despite resuscitation attempts. He was not one of my patients and I saw the nurse phoning his relatives to ask them to come in. I guessed she didn't tell them what had happened. A little later, the man's wife and her sister arrived and the nurse took them into the sister's office to tell them the bad news. I could see the light shining on the three figures in contrast to the darkened ward, like a painting by Edward Hopper.

Suddenly, there was a scream, high, harsh and penetrating with a hoarse rattling in the throat. I looked up, shocked. It was the sort of cry that demanded immediate attention. In the office, the man's wife had fallen to the floor and seemed to be convulsing as she screamed. Her sister was bent over her, sobbing loudly. In a while they were ushered away so that they would not upset the other patients. There was talk of different cultural norms. Staff and patients looked a little shocked as if the man's wife might be dangerous; there was a sense of relief when she left.

But this scream was real, a raw expression of her love and her grief for her husband. I wonder, then, where that scream is in those who receive such news quietly? Of course, such things *are* culturally conditioned. However, I wonder further why it is that Edvard Munch's painting, *The Scream*, is such a ubiquitous image in Western society. The haunting image of a ghostly man, his mouth wide-open, his eyes staring, his hands holding his face, has been reproduced thousands of times. Behind him, two tall figures are walking along the same boardwalk (or is it a bridge?) while a lurid orange sky looks down on a dark headland and a bay reflecting the same vivid colour. Who or what has induced such terror in him? To me, its popularity suggests that we all know that place, though we may not be in touch with it consciously. Perhaps there are times when nothing less will do. At traditional Irish funerals, for example, professional wailers were hired to keen on behalf of the family for their loss. In the same vein, the Biblical descriptions of mourners wearing sackcloth and ashes, and tearing their hair, makes sense, a sort of bodily equivalent of a scream.

There is a fairy tale about the daughter and seven sons of a king. His wife died and he remarried; as is often the way in these stories, his new queen was both wicked and a witch. She hated her stepchildren and she put a curse on the seven sons. She turned them into ravens. She told her stepdaughter that if she did not speak for three years, three months, three weeks and three days, the enchantment would be lifted from them and they would become human again. Much chance *that* would happen. But this faithful sister princess, who was also a grieving daughter, set a seal on her lips and, year after year, remained silent even though she married and had children. Her brothers would fly down to visit her and support her in her terrible task. But there came a time when she could no longer bear the weight of carrying this silence and she went out into the country and found a deep, deep hole that went far down into the Earth. She put her head down into the hole and screamed and howled and screamed again, on and on. And the Earth heard her and took her keening and kept it within her, as might a mother with her child, so that no sound of it was heard above the ground. The girl returned home and never spoke again till the three years, three months, three weeks and three days were up and her brothers were freed from the spell and they were reunited. The wicked queen, of course, came to a bad end.

Chapter 6

Healing

Imagine a broken violin. The strings have snapped, the bridge, the neck and the scroll cracked and the sounding box has caved in. A violinmaker mends it, spending hundreds of hours painstakingly reconstructing it. This is curing. A violinist takes up his remade violin and plays it. What was once lifeless comes to life. This is healing.

I got some inkling of this when I was working at St Christopher's Hospice. One day, as I climbed the stairs leading up to the wards, I heard the sound of music in the distance. I reached the ward where it was coming from and pushed open the swing doors. The volume of sound doubled. Two violinists from the Yehudi Menuhin School were standing in the middle of the ward. One was playing a Bach partita. It was one of those moments. I had been feeling distracted and scattered. Then, in a moment, my whole attention was centred on the music and its player. I felt myself coming alive – there is no other word for it – as I took in the sounds. It was entrancing. The notes sounded cool, liquid, like patterned rain. The whole ward was still and music filled it. They played for a quarter of an hour or so, then took up their music and stands and quietly left to go to another ward. For a while afterwards the ward seemed imbued with a silent afterglow. The patients continued to be ill; some were close to dying. But, for a little, the suffering on the ward seemed transformed.

At our centre, in our soul, we are all whole, a word with the same root as healing. But somehow, as we live our lives, we become disconnected from this place. We are assailed by some trauma that is too much for us to bear and we close down the life in us in order to survive. It becomes encysted, like an egg surrounded by a tough, thick, leathery shell. This can even be enacted literally at a physical level in the form of muscle tension patterns around the body: a clenched jaw, tense neck muscles causing headaches, or abdominal muscles protectively contracted, a kind of body armouring to use a phrase coined by the psychoanalyst, Wilhelm Reich. In short, we freeze.

Healing is like life returning to our frozen self – whether this be our body, our psyche or, indeed, both. When Joan and I were working in a mining village in Northern Canada, we used to go out to see the Churchill River. It was a short drive in a 4x4 along a dirt track which threaded its way through the endless pine forest. The air temperature was -20°C. Deep snow on the ground lightened the dark green of the conifers. There was a single-track bridge made of steel with metal grilles for paving which made a clanking sound when cars drove over them. At first the river was covered with thick ice topped by a blanket of snow, but, as spring advanced and the air temperature rose above freezing, the ice began to crack and then to break off in huge, thick chunks, some the size of a London bus. These were slowly carried away by the dark waters of the river which had continued to flow unseen underneath their icy tomb. At first, the massive lumps bumped into and over each other forming log, or rather ice, jams. It seemed impossible that they would ever free themselves. But, as they slowly melted, a tipping point would arrive and two ice leviathans would suddenly shift and slip apart. Soon the pieces of ice had shrunk to the size of a small car, then the size of a table, and then, in a few weeks, the ice had gone and spring flowers and leaf buds opened in response to the warmth of the sun, while billions of midges prepared to hatch, ready to descend on unsuspecting fishermen.

For us humans, unfreezing can be a painful inner process. I remember times I have woken at night and found my arm numb and paralysed because I had been sleeping on it. I had some inkling of what it felt like to have had a stroke. I would have to pick up my paralysed arm with my other hand to move it in order to allow the strength slowly to come back. In parallel, feeling would begin to return, at first like a flooding of warmth and cold and then intense, painful tingling. Perhaps this gives some idea of what it is like when our frozen psyche comes to life again. We rediscover painful feelings we had long ago buried. Of course this can seem at first like a setback. Actually it may be just the opposite – a sign of healing.

This, however, often needs to be a gradual process. As the ice within us melts, we find some traumatic memory that surfaces and unfreezes. We begin to feel the feelings that we had numbed in the past to protect ourselves. We find ways of addressing the pain. Perhaps we talk to a friend or see a therapist. Slowly our distress eases. Healing has taken place. We feel better. For some this may be enough. For others it is not. As their coldness within melts further, another memory comes to the fore and they go through another cycle. This is a process that may happen repeatedly – for example in those with developmental trauma – as layer after layer of ice melts and entombed traumatic past episodes appear. And, at last, at the centre, at the heart, is the first, the primal wound, which is in essence a failure of love. The task for those who have been thus traumatised is to rediscover this love.

Psychotherapy is often called the 'talking cure'. But for this kind of layered suffering, where memories may not be easily accessible, words may not be enough. The body holds the key; the body remembers. Even in the first years of life, the body holds 'implicit' memories which are not consciously recalled but surface as unexplained physical and psychological symptoms, sometimes years later. Working with bodily sensations, interrogating the language of the body, brings movement and change. We know this idiom instinctively: we have a gut feeling; our heart feels heavy; we feel choked; we have a lump in our throat. And, as we give our body attention, it – and we – begin to flow.

We usually take very little notice of the way our bodies flow. We take it for granted that our blood streams healthily in an endless circle, that air flows in and out of our lungs, that compression waves flow smoothly down our guts moving their contents on. But should something go wrong we know all about it. Obstructions of the bladder, the gut, the coronary arteries or the gall bladder cause, at the very least, intense pain and may be a threat to life itself. I remember so often seeing the intense relief on patients' faces when their particular obstruction was cleared.

Although it may not seem obvious, the healthy brain flows too. Here is how the neurophysiologist Charles Sherrington described the brain waking:

> The great topmost sheet of the mass, that where hardly a light had twinkled or moved, becomes now a sparkling field of rhythmic flashing points with trains of travelling sparks hurrying hither and thither. The brain is waking and with it the mind is returning. It is as if the Milky Way entered upon some cosmic dance. Swiftly the head mass becomes an enchanted loom where millions of flashing shuttles weave a dissolving pattern, always a meaningful pattern though never an abiding one; a shifting harmony of subpatterns.
> (Sherrington 1942)

We need only tune into our thoughts, memories and emotions to experience first-hand how our psyche flows from one experience to another. Indeed our minds are so active that frustrated meditators trying to still their mind have used metaphors such as a tree full of chattering monkeys to describe this ceaseless mental activity. It is when our psyche becomes mired in depression that we realise the importance of flow. Contrast the grey, leaden weight of melancholia to the times we are so completely absorbed in some task that time flows by without our realising it, and we find that an hour has passed seemingly in minutes. It's like comparing a swamp with a free-flowing stream.

So what do masters of different spiritual traditions have to say about how to live our lives, and so how to live healthily? One theme keeps recurring. It is about treating all life, all living – including our body, emotions and mind – all action, all that happens to us, including illness, as sacred. This is not some flight of fancy. They mean it. Hard as it is, they practise it.

Nicolas Herman was born into a poor peasant family in Lorraine in 1614. As a soldier he was involved in the bloody Thirty Years War and was seriously wounded, leaving him with a period of intense emotional distress, a limp and chronic, severe, leg pain. He decided to become a Carmelite in Paris, taking the name Brother Lawrence. He developed a simple personal philosophy which he called the practice of the presence of God; it has surprising similarities to Buddhist meditation. He was considered so remarkable that, despite his humble rank, senior church dignitaries would visit him for advice. One contemporary observed:

> In the greatest hurry of business in the kitchen, he still preserved his recollection and heavenly-mindedness. He was never hasty nor loitering, but did each thing in its season, with an even, uninterrupted composure and tranquillity of spirit. "The time of business," said he, "does not with me differ from the time of prayer; and in the noise and clatter of my kitchen, while several persons are at the same time calling for different things, I possess God in as great tranquillity as if I were on my knees before the Blessed Sacrament."
> (Brother Lawrence 2006, p. 16)

We, too, can give the same attention and care to how we live our lives in even the simplest and most down to earth of ways. The Vietnamese Buddhist monk, Thich Nhat Hanh, for example, speaks in his books of the importance of mindfulness of ordinary everyday actions – eating a tangerine or washing the dishes mindfully or walking in the country. Every act whether sacred or apparently profane is an opportunity to awake. Martin Luther described how he received divine inspiration once as he sat on the toilet. Everything is grist for this mill.

Could this also apply to the experience of illness? The Buddha is reputed to have died of food poisoning, seemingly such an ignoble end for such a remarkable person. But even as he lay dying he was absorbed in a meditative state. He did not treat his illness, painful though it was, as his enemy. For a time it was simply part of his existence. His awareness encompassed his illness rather than the other way round.

Of course it is well and good that an enlightened one can take such a course. But what about the unenlightened rest of us who struggle with the fears of pain, illness and death? I believe one answer is in the care that surrounds us – or not – when we are ill. Care is such a widely used word that it has lost some of its original power. One derivation comes from *caritas*, the Latin word for love, which we still use when we say: "I care about you." Sometimes, though, our care is efficient but lacking in love.

For many women, labour takes place in a climate of technology. Painful electrodes are attached to the baby's head to monitor its heart rate; contractions are also monitored; drips may be set up to expedite labour; drugs to contract the uterus are administered as soon as the baby is born, babies slither out into a world of painfully dazzling lights, frightening noises and cold air, and the cord which connected them for so long and so intimately to their mother is cut straight away. If they don't breathe immediately, they may be slapped and even have a breathing tube inserted into their trachea and oxygen is blown into their lungs. No wonder many babies scream so. They are overwhelmed by distress and terror.

Does it have to be like this? Perhaps not. Emergencies do, of course, require interventions such as caesarean sections, and yet... I remember being deeply moved when I watched a film by Dr Frederick Leboyer entitled *Birth Without Violence*. As I watched it, I recalled that nurses caring for the dying are sometimes called midwives. In a quiet room with dimmed lights, Dr Leboyer's hands were seen gently massaging a woman's pregnant abdomen and indirectly the baby inside. His movements were calm and slow and when the woman gave birth she didn't cry out. These were healing hands I thought to myself. Dr Leboyer received the baby and he carefully placed her on her mother's naked abdomen, skin to skin. The baby cried out as she took her first breaths but this quickly abated to a few quiet whimpers. He tenderly massaged the baby's head, its back, its legs, while her mother supported her with one of her hands. These were totally new sensations for the baby. She continually opened and closed her fingers. Blinking, she looked up at the faces around her – again a new sensation. Only when the umbilical cord had stopped pulsing did Dr Leboyer cut the cord. A little later he placed her in a bath of warm water, continuing the massaging all the time. This *was* familiar to her and she relaxed and became quieter. She still moved her arms a little and, at one stage, discovered she could suck her fingers. Later, out of the water, she rested her head in Dr Leboyer's hands. Her face was completely calm, her eyes lightly closed. It looked like the face of a person deep in contemplation. Newborn babies aren't supposed to be able to smile but she did.

And what about the midwifery of dying? Certainly those close to death may experience fear, panic, terror even, which demand containment, just as in childbirth. The same rhythms of quietness, touch, breathing and opening to a new reality apply:

I pass by a hospice single room. The door is slightly ajar. The patient lies quietly asleep in bed; the lights are low. Her husband sits at her bedside holding her hand.

A doctor is visiting a patient at home. Carefully and gently she examines him. It is as though she is having a conversation with his body. His stomach hurts. She takes extra care not to cause him pain. Later, his wife massages his hands and feet, comforting him. Earlier that day a nurse had visited and helped his wife to reposition him in his bed. All through the day, then, hands are laid on him. He is calmed by their contact.

A woman is close to death and sleeping. She wakes; her eyes open wide with surprise. She tells her family sitting by her bed that she can see members of her family who have died. She is looking into another world. It is a good experience for her. Some of her living family believe her, some don't and think she is confused.

A woman sits with her husband just as he is dying. The intervals between his breaths lengthen. At last, some eighty years after he took in his first breath as a newborn baby, he breathes out one last breath and his body becomes still. His heart ceases to beat. His wife, in tears, gets up and embraces him, one long, last embrace, pressing her face against his cheek as if this could somehow keep him with her. After a while she feels that he is no longer there. Something – she knows not what – has gone from his body.

There is also this: if you even attempt to treat all life as holy, then others may in return see the holiness, the wholeness, in you. Possibilities are born: loneliness might just give way to love, emptiness to fullness, despair to hope, fear to refuge. Light pierces the dark night that our souls have endured. What else would we live for?

The Eagle and the Mountain

I got to know Bill Ellis while he was writing a book about the story of his illness. (Ellis 1981) I was working as a junior doctor at St Joseph's Hospice in 1979. Bill lived in St Patrick's Wing, a part of the hospice then set aside for patients with long-term illnesses. In 1968, in his early thirties, he developed encephalitis which led to quadriplegia, paralysis of all four limbs. How did he feel after waking from his coma?

> But my inability to do anything, even to move a muscle, made me deeply depressed. Tears flood out as I tried to move and could achieve nothing. No sound, no movement, and inside me an emptiness that was terrible. Although now I may have been better than when I was in the black world of the unconscious, my state seemed to me to be of a vegetable – a vegetable with feelings that seemed only of depression and frustration. I think this must have been the lowest point of all in my illness, for the only moments when I was awake I was in a fog of melancholy and despair. (p. 23)

His wife, Dorothy, was a constant support to him. Together they worked out a way of communicating – blinking: one blink for yes and two for no. A first small victory. He describes having a nasogastric tube for feeding and a catheter for urinary incontinence. Sometimes, overcome by his plight and these indignities, he would wail and scream inarticulately. However, speech therapy helped him produce a variety of different sounds that could be used towards communication rather than only a raw keening. For months, though, he continued to experience waves of deep depression. Then came another breakthrough – a visit home for a night and then every weekend. Little by little, other achievements followed as he gained better head and finger movements – reading, using an electronic typewriter with a control attached to his head, being able to articulate some slurred words, driving an electric wheelchair and feeding himself. Painting, using armrests so that his fingers holding the brush were just over the paper, was a particular pleasure. The book movingly portrays his immense efforts to regain his life. After stays at several rehabilitation centres and hospitals, he was transferred to St Joseph's Hospice in 1974.

Every time I visited him, he was smiling and welcoming. Communication was a slow business, but Bill was very patient and determined. He continued his visits home, his painting and writing. It didn't matter that he took many times longer than an able-bodied person. The publication of his book was a testament to his tenacity. He wanted to live his life and he wasn't going to let his illness stop him. He was interviewed by a BBC reporter and he said: "… I accept life as it is, grateful that I am so lucky in so many ways… so very many ways…" (p. 180) How many of us could say that if we had to contend daily with the sorts of difficulties that were his lot?

There is a very characteristic photograph of him in the book. (p. 160) He is sitting in his wheelchair, smiling broadly with his hands folded across his lap. On the wall behind him are two of his paintings, which I remember seeing when I used to visit him. The first shows the head of an eagle. The other shows a landscape with mountains, forests and a lake, painted in great detail – just the place for an eagle. At first sight these seem poignant. Bill couldn't walk and would never see an eagle in the wild. I think though these were paintings of his soulscape, his inner world where nothing was barred, where he could climb mountains, where his imagination could take flight.

In Native American spirituality, the eagle signifies endurance, strength and vision. An eagle flying east represents life renewal. It seems appropriate that Bill chose to paint this bird. Here was an ordinary person in extraordinary circumstances who experienced a dark night of the soul and who, out of this, found a way of creating and living a fulfilling life for himself.

Do Mention the War

My uncle, an officer in the Australian army during the Second World War, was captured by the Japanese and worked on the construction of the infamous Burma (or Death) railway which killed 16,000 Allied prisoners of war and 90,000 Asian labourers. He survived this and was transported in what was known as a hellship to Japan to be interned in a prisoner of war camp. He was lucky to survive this journey since some of the hellships were sunk by Allied aircraft bombing – the pilots did not know the transport ships held Allied servicemen. He even survived the brutal conditions of the camp – just. Though he was a big man he weighed six stone when his camp was liberated. Afterwards, he never talked about his experiences.

This is one story among several of my family's experiences of war. Just about everybody will have had some such connection – as soldiers, as prisoners of war, as mourners of family members killed or as members of a race or culture experiencing systematic attempts at annihilation.

Like so many others I feel passionately that these stories should not be forgotten. In psychotherapy, individuals find, and make meaning from, their stories and in this way heal. It is the same for nations. Denial and repression is not healthy for individuals, nor is it for nations. It still happens, though, and that includes the 'good guy' nations.

An example of this is what used to be called 'shell shock' in the First World War. Large numbers of troops experienced this. Many were labelled 'weak', 'inferior' or 'cowardly'. Some were executed for desertion; most likely they were just trying to escape the intolerable and overwhelming hell that was the lot of soldiers in the trenches. In hindsight, we can recognise these as cases of post-traumatic stress disorder, now accepted medically as a psychological injury occasioned here by the extreme stress of combat. Somehow, though, after the end of the First World War, 'shell shock' lapsed into obscurity and it was only with the onset of the Second World War that armies were forced, once more, to acknowledge the reality of this condition. The Vietnam, Iraq and Afghan wars, with their steady fallout of psychologically traumatised soldiers, have had the unintended effect of preventing a repeat of the earlier whitewashes.

For those of us who have not been in a war, it is hard to imagine the effect on those in front-line combat. We watch the news or documentaries or war films but these can only give a hint of the effect of actually being there, of the deafening sounds of bombs, gun and rocket fire, the screaming of the wounded, the smells of blood and dirt and fear, the sight of friends blown up by a mine, the dry mouth and pounding heart, and of eyes searching restlessly for the enemy. Many soldiers spend years living with horrifying nightmares, flashbacks and extreme emotions and feel they just have to put up with their distress; they may drink or take drugs in an effort to numb or forget their pain. There are effective therapeutic methods available and among these is – to mention the war. They need to be able to speak about the unspeakable, put words to it, to be heard, to be able to reconstruct a meaningful story within which to contain the dreadfulness of their experiences within a secure milieu and, a step at a time, to heal.

Some of the patients I have looked after have experienced wars directly. I remember one old Polish man who had been in a German prison camp during the Second World War. He was a quiet man built like a small bear with thinning short white hair and a greyish-white pallor to his skin. His English was strongly accented and difficult to understand. He had a room of his own, one of twelve on the ward. As his cancer advanced, his hold on everyday reality slowly slipped. Confusion grew. One day we found him wandering around the ward and peering into the other rooms. In one of these was a woman who had just died.

Apart from a subdued restlessness he appeared apparently less troubled than we were about what he had seen. We talked with him in his room. He had developed a delusional world all of his own. He was back in his prison camp. The staff were the warders. The rooms were like the prison huts. He wasn't surprised to see a dead person as this happened regularly in the camp – whether they had died through starvation or execution.

I was horrified, not only because he had gone through such a terrible experience during the war, but also because it had stayed with him and, triggered by his final illness, had even invaded his outer reality. In hindsight, I can recognise that greyish-white skin as most likely a mark of a chronic, frozen traumatic state. At least, though, we were able to do something: we were able to ease his psychotic state with medications, granting him some peace before he died.

When my father was with the Allied Forces as they swept through Germany at the end of the Second World War, he was tasked, as part of the medical corps, with going into liberated prison and concentration camps to provide urgent medical care for the inmates, a remarkable experience. He was overseeing the provision of the life-saving food and water, vitamins and medicines that these starving prisoners desperately needed. It must have been wonderful to watch people weighing five stone gradually heal, putting on weight and coming back to life. It must have been touching to see their joy at being free again and their gratitude to their liberators.

And yet there were some who had gone too far along the road to their death. Even with the necessary food and drugs, they died. "You could see it in their eyes," my father said. Eyes that were like extinguished candles, empty. When faced with overwhelming, long-continued cruelty and neglect, this was their last escape. Their body shut down. A primitive part of the autonomic nervous system (one we share with reptiles) was activated which slowed and then stopped their heart. A mercy, really.

The capacity we humans have for inflicting pain on one another is extraordinary. It is only matched by our capacity for compassion. So – please – do mention the war. We need to remember and learn.

Two Men and a Dog Called Marjorie

I'm looking at a faded black and white photograph. It has captured a key moment of discovery in medicine. It shows two men and a dog standing outside a building on a sunny day. The man on the right is about thirty but looks older. He wears round spectacles and a grey laboratory coat; he has rolled the sleeves up to his elbows. He leans forward slightly and is smiling. The man on the left is much younger, in his early twenties, with a shy smile. He is dressed in a white shirt and tie (which is blowing in the wind) and dark trousers. His right hand is on his hip and, like his companion, his sleeves are rolled up. Between them is a small slender dog, with long, flopping ears, white muzzle, chest and legs, and dark torso and head.

The picture was taken in 1921 on the roof of the Medical Building at the University of Toronto. The older man was Dr Frederick Banting and the younger was a medical student called Charles Best. They were looking for a treatment for diabetes and had found that a pancreatic extract, insulin, kept diabetic dogs alive. One, called Marjorie, lived for seventy days. Buoyed by their success, they gave insulin to a 14 year old boy dying of diabetes; he dramatically recovered within days. They published their results in 1922. What was once a lethal disease that killed millions could now be controlled by simple injections.

She was about fifteen years old but had been admitted to my medical ward because she was post-pubertal. I was – to say the least – alarmed when I first saw her. She was about as ill as you could be without actually being dead. Her GP thought she was haemorrhaging from her stomach and vomiting up blood. She was unconscious and had what is called the Hippocratic facies, the look of someone with extreme dehydration, which Hippocrates himself first described. Her eyes were sunken with dark shadows encircling them. Her skin was so parched of fluid you could pick up folds of it. Her tongue was thickly coated and literally dry. Her pulse was fast and thready, her blood pressure almost too low to record. Her whole body looked shrunken.

And yet, despite this, I could see her good looks as well. She was tall, black, with an Afro hairstyle and a beautiful face.

We soon discovered the cause of her illness. One of the nurses had tested her urine and found it to be strongly positive to glucose. She was in a diabetic coma. It turned out that what her GP had thought was blood was actually redcurrant juice she had been drinking. We swung into emergency action with replacement intravenous fluids, electrolytes and insulin. Even so, I doubted whether she would live.

I spoke to her father. He was in his forties, a round-faced African man of medium height. I felt I had to be candid and warn him of the risk that she might die. I still remember his worried face and the way he looked down and clicked his tongue. I didn't know whether I had transgressed cultural boundaries in speaking so openly and yet I felt, too, that it was essential to prepare him for the worst.

We worked hard on resuscitating her and, to my relief, she survived. Her blood glucose level slowly returned from its stratospheric heights to normal levels. She remained unconscious into the next day and then gradually woke up. The day after, she was up and walking around. I was astonished at how quickly she recovered. I watched as her father's expression changed gradually from heaviness and worry to relief and delight. His daughter had returned to him. As for me, I was more than happy.

The Dunkirk Arm

As pre-clinical medical students, we attended lectures in an old wooden auditorium with stepped rows of wooden benches and desktops. These were angled so that they formed a curve. The worn wooden desktops were incised or inked with generations of student graffiti. From our place in the gods, we looked down at our lecturer far below. The scene was reminiscent of the centuries' old medical lecture theatres which featured a dissection table completely surrounded by steeply stepped circular walkways and railings over which leaned medical students watching the dissections taking place below and listening to the expert commentary of their professor of anatomy.

Our lectures were not often memorable, but there was one I still remember. It was a talk given by our anatomy professor, a small, earnest, grey-haired woman who habitually dressed in a tweed skirt, grey blouse and sensible flat shoes. She showed us an X-ray of the upper arm of a soldier who had been badly wounded during the evacuation of Dunkirk in the Second World War. His upper arm had been severely traumatised by a bomb blast. Not only was the soft tissue damaged, but also his humerus – the bone had been shattered into dozens of fragments so that the shaft of the bone could no longer be traced on the X-ray. All that was visible were the random splinters and chips of bone. No operation was possible here. The soft tissues of the arm were left to heal of their own accord. She then showed us another X-ray taken some weeks later in which we could see the fragments of bone regrowing and coalescing. Eventually they formed a healing egg-shaped lump of bone that gradually remodelled itself to form a new normal bone shaft.

I was astonished at this extreme example of the healing power of the body. We are used to seeing this with cuts or even surgical wounds, but this trauma seemed so grave that bone healing could surely not have taken place – and yet it did. This was one time when I was shaken out of my habitual way of seeing the world so that I suddenly realised just how remarkable the healing process is. In its own small way it was a moment of enlightenment.

The Worst Tube Journey in the World

It's strange how some memories stand out among a blur of forgetting. During our medical student pharmacology module we attended a series of lectures on different classes of drugs. One of the lecturers, a small man in his forties, balding and with swept back dark hair kept in place by some nameless gel, was memorable for being able to hold our attention, or mine at least. He had the gift of speaking clearly and making connections. We understood. He had worked on the initial clinical trials of a drug called frusemide, a powerful diuretic. As part of this, he decided one day to give himself an injection of this drug and observe the effect on his output of urine. Nothing happened. He waited a couple of hours and then, disappointed with its lack of outcome, as it were, he decided to go home. Halfway along the longest stretch of London underground tube line between two stops, the frusemide acted – and fast. He only just made it to the next station and was forced, to his embarrassment, to pee huge volumes of dilute urine in the corner of the Tube platform. The manufacturers had promised a 'torrential diuresis'. Now he knew the truth of this from personal experience.

A few years later, I was working as a house physician when an elderly woman was admitted to my ward around midnight. She had suffered a massive heart attack and had gone into severe congestive cardiac failure. Her lungs had become waterlogged. Every breath was a huge effort and her respirations crackled from the air bubbling through her fluid-filled bronchi. A chest X-ray showed a sort of white snowstorm almost obliterating the normally dark lungs. She was slowly suffocating in her secretions.

Things were different then. We didn't have a coronary care unit. There was only myself and the night nurse, who had to look after the whole ward, and an electrocardiogram to read off the patient's heart rhythms. Apart from other cardiac drugs, I gave her a large dose of frusemide intravenously to relieve her water-logged lungs. In a short while she began to pass urine – and then a lot of urine. Over hours her breathing gradually quietened and eased and a further chest X-ray showed that the pale clouds obscuring her lungs were in retreat. On admission, she was close to dying. By the morning, she was on the road to recovery.

It is a scene I have seen repeated so many times and one that has always moved me even though it is so commonplace. There is something extraordinarily satisfying in being able to turn on such a powerful pharmacological tap to such good effect. Severe breathlessness is one of the worst symptoms you can have. It's not surprising that patients are so grateful. It is like being rescued from drowning. The pharmacology of the drug is interesting enough but it's nothing like the excitement of watching a form of resurrection taking place.

Feel-See

When we were in Hawaii, Joan and I met an old Hawaiian man, a respected Elder. We were fortunate because Hawaiians understandably don't wish to talk about their culture with passing tourists just looking for a photo opportunity. When we met him, he was sitting under a tree shading him from the sun, while members of his family were nearby. He told us stories about his life and my main memory is of feeling goose bumps, shivers and excitement as he spoke. This was soul talk.

We were asking him about something we had been told that shamans use, a way of looking. In the West, we tend to concentrate on one thing when we look. Shamans, however, may do the opposite. They deliberately allow their vision to go out of focus and so make space for their whole field of view in their awareness. We tend automatically to do something similar if we gaze out to sea. They then allow their vision to be drawn to whatever catches their eye. It's a way of allowing intuition to guide you to whatever is significant in front of you. Perhaps this is what psychotherapists do when, following Freud's lead, they let their attention hover evenly as they look at their client.

"Ah yes," the Elder said. "Feel-see." He went on to explain. It is part of Hawaiian culture and he described instances. When he was young, if he was going out fishing with his brother, they would look out to sea in this widely aware way to see where the fishing might be good, but they would also feel what they saw. Sometimes, one of them would say they shouldn't go out past such and such an island, there was a shark around. If they did pass by there, there would be the shark. And he went on to explain how their small boat might be at risk, circled by sharks, attracted by the fish bait in the water.

We were fascinated. I thought of how often, as a doctor, I would concentrate all my attention on one part of the body that was ailing. There's a need, too, to sit back, and take in the whole of the person in front of you, to feel-see them. If your attention is intuitively drawn by something seemingly irrelevant – a faded shirt, a facial twitch, scuffed worn shoes, restlessness – it may be worth taking note of it. It could just be relevant.

The Hidden City

I was working as a trainee general practitioner and had been seconded to work in a practice on the edge of Dartmoor. My accommodation was the local cottage hospital where I found I had the run of the top floor while the patients were in a series of rooms on the ground floor. It was the sort of place that I liked: small, quiet, unhurried; almost in a time warp.

One day, my trainer said we were going to visit a hospital up in the hills. We left the little town and wound our way up a deserted narrow road with rocky inclines on either side. There was a slight mist in the air and, as we climbed higher, the vegetation became that of the moorlands: gorse, grass cropped short by sheep and wild ponies, and a few stunted trees. We came at last to an entrance on our right and drove up a long, winding driveway flanked by trees. As we drove, my trainer told me that this was an old TB isolation hospital which was no longer used as such because of the advent of curative antibiotics for this condition. Now, just one of the wards housed a group of people with learning difficulties. We rounded a corner and there was the hospital. It was huge with a series of long wards, operating theatre suites, an administration block and staff accommodation, all laid out in spacious, hilly grounds among lawns and ornamental flowering bushes. There was an eerie quietness to the place. He showed me around. There were the operating theatres. These used to be in constant use carrying out thoracoplasties, an operation to collapse the upper part of the chest and so deprive the TB bacteria within of oxygen. I had come across a few patients in the past who had had this procedure and it was very disfiguring, causing a sort of artificial curvature of the spine. Now the theatres were empty, dusty and unused. We walked through them and I saw a few items of surgical equipment left around haphazardly. There was none of the antiseptic smell of operating theatres in action; rather, with the windows closed, it smelled stale. It had a ghostly abandoned air. Outside there was a long veranda where patients used to sit and enjoy the sun. Now, all that was left were a few empty, rickety chairs.

We moved down the hill to the wards. They were long and high-ceilinged and had high doors at each end which would be opened, summer and winter, as it was believed that fresh air helped the healing process for TB. I was told that this applied even when it was snowing. There used to be carefully graded exercise regimes and woe betide the patient who took it upon himself to exercise too much. These were Nightingale wards which had neat rows of beds on each side of the ward. At that time, many of those admitted were, in effect, terminally ill and would have died there. Again I felt the sense of emptiness, of loss and melancholy. It was like exploring ruins.

One of the wards had been divided in half and in one half was the accommodation for inmates with learning difficulties such as Down's syndrome. Suddenly, the place felt alive with their talk and interactions. It was like a small enclave set in a wilderness. My trainer had to see one of the residents and, when he had finished examining him and prescribing, we went on our way.

I felt as though I had encountered a piece of history. I was still haunted by the atmosphere as we drove down the Dartmoor valley and I was left wondering at this example, firstly of how prevalent and feared TB was – as much as cancer is nowadays – and, secondly, of what an extraordinary effect the advent of antibiotics had, enough to render places such as this, with their strange and desperate therapies, obsolete. This is, surely, a dramatic example of the advance of medical science, and I thought of how treatment for TB is so often taken for granted nowadays. My ghost hospital was a reminder of how it used to be.

Beginner's Luck

The way that hospices first made the news was through controlling previously uncontrollable pain. It seemed like a miracle in an area that had been fraught with fear and denial. I remember the first person I treated using hospice principles. I was working in general practice then and had been called to see Robert at home because he had severe back pain from spinal cancer. Sometime earlier he had developed weakness of the legs due to pressure on the spine from the cancer; he was lucky that an emergency operation restored the use of his legs. He lived alone in a large bungalow. It was getting dark as I drove into his gravelled driveway – it was a wet, cold, late autumn evening and this seemed to mirror what I would find when I met him. I rang the bell. When he opened the door, he looked unwell. He was restless, with the grey pallor that some people with severe pain get, and he was desperate. As he showed me his wide range of analgesics, he informed me with a mixture of anger and resignation that none of his medicines worked. With the enthusiasm of a convert, I explained how I would treat him. In fact he didn't need new medications, just a more effective use of what he already had. This, I was to discover, is one of the secrets of good symptom control – attention to detail, even to the extent of writing out exactly what medication is to be taken, and when. The next day I returned, wondering what I would find. When I rang the doorbell, a very different Robert, looking much better, flung the door open, seized my hand and couldn't stop shaking it. His pain had almost disappeared and he thanked me over and over again. I was delighted and rather bewildered. It seemed too good to be true. And what pleasure I had in seeing his relief that the dreaded pain, that seemingly invincible monster, had retreated.

This sort of story is common in hospice care but it was new

for me then. I'd previously looked after many people with pain that remained difficult to control. 'Heartsink', or perhaps 'heartsunk' was not a bad description for how I used to feel. I had been converted to using hospice principles in the space of 24 hours.

A Spring of Water

I am sitting on a long, weathered, white-painted bench, one of many in rows. I am facing a cliff, in which is set a shallow grotto, partly in shade as evening draws near. To the right, there is a large candleholder containing many circles of thin candles each two to three feet high rising in tiers to the single candle at the top, about 12 feet above the ground. Their flames flicker in the slight breeze. Above the candles, in a tree-fringed niche in the rocks, is a statue of a woman in a white robe. I get up and take my place in the line of people entering the grotto on the right, following the curving contours of the rocks, and then coming out again on the left. In the floor of this tiny cave is a thick glass pane, brightly lit. As I look down I can see a spring of water gushing from a cleft in the rocks. I walk round the grotto and watch the other people ahead. Each one touches the rocky wall with their hand or with some object like a handkerchief. To my amazement, the rough stone has been worn to a glassy smoothness by millions of people, year upon year, doing the same. I come out again and sit down. Sometime later, events take a surreal turn. Cardinal Basil Hume[3] appears and walks through the grotto. No one seems to notice him and he walks off again by himself. No security. No cameras. No journalists. It must have been a blessed relief for him to be able to do this.

Nearby, the water from the spring has been channelled into bathhouses. People come there to immerse themselves in the water and avail themselves of its healing properties. Earlier that day, I decided to take the plunge. There was a changing room where I exchanged my clothes for the sort of bathing costume they wore in the 1940s. It was definitely the wet look – the black clinging material moulded itself to my pelvic contours more intimately than I would have liked; the waistband reached my navel. Also changing was a man in his forties, there with his two sons, who came here every year following the death of his wife from cancer – he and his wife had gained much support from the time he brought her here. I noticed, as he changed, that he had holes in his Y-fronts. Not enough money, I wondered, or perhaps struggling to bring his children up single-handed and no time for his own needs. I felt touched and saddened.

When it was my turn, I pushed aside a curtain and saw a large bath, about 6 feet square with steps leading down into it. Two cheerful men with rolled-up sleeves were waiting in the crystal clear water. At my assistants' bidding I stepped down into the waters. They explained what they would do. They began praying in French. As they drew to a close, they asked me to hold my nose. They firmly but gently took hold of my arms and immersed me backwards. I remember thinking that the water did not feel particularly cold, though it had come straight from some chilly underground source. It also had a very smooth quality – I could slide my finger and thumb across each other more easily than I could, say, in a shower at home. I left feeling – cool.

When I came out of the bathhouses, I walked past a long water pipe running from the grotto along the face of the cliffs and parallel to the ground. At regular intervals, there were taps and crowds of people were drinking the water, splashing their faces, and collecting some in bottles. A particularly tough-looking group of Spaniards were pushing their way through to the front. No politeness here. They meant business. They had five-gallon plastic containers. What did they want with all those litres, I wondered.

The open spaces nearby are crowded with thousands of people sweltering in the warm sun. Some appear able-bodied, some limping, some walk with crutches and some are being pushed along in wheelchairs. I become acutely aware of the purpose of this place as one where huge numbers of the sick, the dying and their families come, looking for help of a different kind. Here, they are centre stage and respected. I talk to one woman in her thirties. She has leukaemia and is in remission following chemotherapy. She has come to give thanks. She knows she may get a recurrence, but she is grateful for the present reprieve.

That night, there is a procession. It is perhaps one-third of a mile in length, and this is a quiet night. Each participant holds a candle. I watch from the vantage point of some steps to gain a better view. It is like seeing a huge river of light stream slowly forwards, accompanied by a continuous background of singing. They come to a large open area where the river spills into a wide circular lake of light shimmering with the points of the candle flames. I am mesmerised by the beauty of something so simple.

Lourdes. Such a strange phenomenon, you might think. Who would want to travel hundreds, even thousands, of miles in the discomfort of planes, trains or buses, when they might be so ill that only lying down on a stretcher will do. And it's not just Christians. Muslims travel to Mecca, Hindus to the enormous Ardh Kumbh Mela religious festival on the Ganges, host to tens of millions of pilgrims.

Religion comes originally from the Latin *re-ligare* meaning to bind together. (Chambers 1988) What I have tried to describe is a binding together of people in the best sense, like a family bound together by ties of love. This sort of religion is visceral, felt, relational, personal and grounded. It does not concern itself much with intellectual abstractions or dogmatic assertions. This applies particularly to ill people who are suffering. Their approach is based on a personal relationship with a divine figure or a saint – Jesus, Mary, Muhammad, Krishna, Ganesh, Buddha, Zarathustra – in whom they put their trust. And if this means they must travel great distances at great cost, personal and financial, in their search for healing, then they will do it.

It's also about finding acceptance of whatever happens, a miracle in itself. I have talked to so many ill people who are caught up – understandably – in fear, sadness, bitterness and despair that it's shocking when I meet someone who just accepts his condition. And remarkable.

I See You

I first saw Edward at home. I liked him immediately, his sincerity, his thoughtfulness and his courage in facing his condition. In his late thirties, he was tall, very thin, with a quiff of thick, blond hair and studious tortoise-shell glasses. He was also very ill and hardly able to get out of his bed. His cancer had spread from its original site in the gut and was beginning to break down, causing changes in the electrolyte balance of his blood. A pity, I thought sadly, that such a young man with so much life in him would soon die. His brother was taking care of him and, when I had explained what I had found, I arranged, with their agreement, for him to be admitted urgently to the hospice.

He told me that he had been using a visualisation technique to counteract his cancer. This had been developed by an American husband and wife couple, the Simontons; he was an oncologist and she a psychologist. Their book, called *Getting Well Again* (Simonton, Matthews-Simonton and Creighton 1986), describing these techniques was a worldwide best-seller. Using one of their exercises, Edward imagined his immune system – his molecular antibodies and protective white cells – as sharks. He would visualise millions of these microscopic predators flooding through his bloodstream, seeking out any cancer cells and destroying them, just as sharks hunt down fish. And then? Why then by the principle of sympathy, the energy, the power, the ferocity of the pitiless sharks flying through the imagined vessels of his mind would be translated to, absorbed by, his immune system which, primed and strengthened, would renew its unceasing attack on the cancer cells.

In the hospice, after we had stabilised his condition, I talked to him about his visualisations. Our conversation went something like this:

I say to him, "Edward." "Yes," he says. "The image-work you've been doing – is it helping much right now?" "No," he says, "it isn't." "So, why not try something a bit different?" "Yes," he says cheerfully not knowing what I'm about to tell him. "Instead of the sharks," I say, "why not try this: First, imagine what your cancer looks like." I can see that's easy for him. He closes his eyes, imagining hard. "It's black," he says (they almost always choose black, I think to myself), "and spiky, a blob." I think: Unexploded mine. I can see his disgust, his anger at his enemy.

"Try this," I say. "Imagine a light, a light shining down from above on to the cancer. Just that; you don't need to do anything about it. Just watch; oh, and the light can be any colour you want." "Yes," he says and goes quiet.

"What's happening, Edward," I ask. He's excited. "It's changing," he says. "The light is affecting the cancer; it's starting to bubble and melt." He keeps watching. I get progress reports: "It's getting smaller," he says. Silence. Then: "It's gone," he concludes, and looks, well – lit-up.

We look at each other, see each other. I'm wondering what is happening here. I'm sharing his excitement but cautious me needs to put a word in. "Look," I say, "this is just an image." "Yes," he says. "It's just an image," I repeat. "It doesn't mean that the cancer's gone." Yes, he understands that. But, for a while, he's on cloud nine. Even if it's *just* an image, he has become re-empowered. That black mine hadn't just attacked his body, it had infiltrated his thoughts, his feelings, even his relationships. Watching it go geed him up no end.

I wondered what would happen next. He carried on being excited and told the nurses all about it as they attended to him. He was content, accepting and Alive-with-a-capital-A. And that's how he continued. He did the light exercise from time to time for himself. You don't often see someone looking so peaceful – and then he died a few days later.

What, died? Shouldn't he have got better? I don't think so. This was about more than his physical state; it was about all the rest of him that had been permeated by the dark crab. It was his release from this that had been important. Of course he was peaceful. He was ready to go. He wasn't cured, but he was surely healed.

My meetings with Edward reminded me of the way Zulus traditionally greet each other: "Sawubona." It means, "I see you," and you're meant to respond: "Ngikhona," meaning "I am here." isn't that wonderful welcome? How could we wish for anything more than to be seen in our dignity, to be seen for who we truly are, and thus to know that we are here, now, in this very moment, feet on the ground, our hearts beating, breathing God's good air. Meditators spend a lifetime practising this.

What is it like to see in this way? It is as if, when you sit down with someone who is ill, even before you say anything, your eyes are saying: "Yes, I do see you; I am taking in who you are, your looks, the way you smile or look sad, your anger, too. I see your clothes, their style, how you're speaking through them, what mood they convey. I see the ways you move, the way you go still when you're frightened, the way your face changes as you talk. I see your laugh and find myself laughing back. I see your questions and your doubts, your anxieties. I see you when you feel strong and the times when you feel weak and downcast. And I see you looking at me, taking me in, watching my reactions, searching to see if you can trust me."

This being seen is, I think, something we want more than anything in the world, and yet, paradoxically, it's something we shy away from. With good reason we defend ourselves, protect our vulnerability. To trust a person enough to let him see you is a privilege that has to be earned. I was touched that Edward extended this trust to me.

The Woman Who Wouldn't Have Her Leg Cut Off

Maud was thin, elderly and anxious, with a thick thatch of hair, dyed chestnut-brown. She had been admitted to a geriatric ward because she had developed gangrene of the toes of her left foot. This was due to narrowing of the arteries supplying her foot and had been aggravated by her being a long-term smoker, which of itself causes arterial constriction.

Day by day the medical team would visit her and inspect her unprepossessing black toes. Conservative measures were not working and the gangrene seemed to be advancing slowly up her foot. There was nothing for it. Maud would have to have an amputation to prevent a fatal spread of the gangrene.

Maud refused – despite considerable pressure on her and a frank explanation of what would happen to her: in summary, that she would die. But Maud held firm. The thought of an operation to remove a part of her anatomy she had lived with all her life was just too much for her.

My consultant then decided to put in place palliative care measures to keep her comfortable until her demise. She would need, he told us, regular morphine every four hours to keep the pain in her foot at bay. She would gradually deteriorate, stop eating, lose weight, stop drinking and then die. Maud, however, refused to play by the rules. She needed morphine only sporadically and continued to eat and drink a little.

Weeks went by and, suddenly, Maud surprised us again. She decided to have the operation after all. The medical team felt she might die under the anaesthetic, but, in fact, she sailed through. A few days later, the physiotherapist was teaching her to use crutches and, though still anxious, she stood up for the first time in many weeks and, very slowly, began to move around her room.

What Maud needed was time. Her fear was so overwhelming to begin with that she could not take in what was being offered to her. Through her refusal, she gave herself enough time for her fear to reduce enough to allow her to come to terms with the loss of her leg. It was no good giving her rational reasons why she needed the operation; her fear was much more deep-seated than that. It had a childlike quality to it, as though she had gone back to a place where she was experiencing the sort of terror that is impervious to adult reasoning. What she needed was an experience of safety, and she inadvertently received this through staying in bed and being cared for by the nurses and given medicines to soothe her pain.

This, of course, was not the intention of the clinical team. She was, perhaps, seen as 'difficult'; there was no time on a busy hospital ward for such time-wasting behaviour, they would have argued. To my mind, the team did the right thing in the end, even if for the wrong reasons.

When I began working in palliative medicine, this need for patients to take time to make decisions was a recurring and important theme. We are none of us machines. We all feel, and it is only natural that we may feel fear when confronting a major illness (or even a minor one with worrying symptoms for that matter). Those of us who are clinicians need to bear this in mind. There is a wonderful photograph in an old copy of the St Christopher's Hospice Annual Review. It shows an old man sitting on the side of his bed with the ward sister sitting beside him and holding a little plastic pot of tablets. The caption simply comments that Bill, the patient, is taking time to decline his drugs.

Pictures in a House

I sometimes think about the many hundreds of homes I have visited as a doctor. I always found that such visits added so much to my understanding of patients and their families; information I could never get simply from taking a medical history. I visited one elderly man several times. What I remember most was a chrome model of a Spitfire on a table in the hallway along with dozens of black and white framed photographs of Second World War planes that neatly lined the walls leading upstairs to his bedroom. No prizes for guessing where his interests and memories lay.

A few of the people I visited were obviously well off. The walls of their houses might be hung with hunting prints, antique paintings, perhaps of ancestors, while china dogs and Chinese vases and clocks sat on mantelpieces and dressers. But what about the less well off, those struggling to make ends meet, living in council houses? Over the years, I grew familiar with the sights and smells of poverty – damp; the odour of boiled cabbages and potatoes and of smoke from cigarettes and the coal fire, the only form of heating in the house; dog smells; and the mustiness of frayed old sofas with collapsed springs. Nevertheless, mostly there was *some* form of decoration in these houses and I noticed certain reproductions of paintings appearing again and again. One of them is called *Wings of Love* by Stephen Pearson. It shows a naked man and woman looking out at a dreamlike, moonlit, calm, night sea while the wings of a huge swan encircle them from above. Another is *Chinese Girl*, or *Green Lady*, by Vladimir Tretchikoff, of which there are many versions. It shows the eponymous Chinese girl, wearing an oriental dress, looking down and to her left, her face serious and unfathomable, her skin varying from green to bronze, her black hair long and her lips rouged. A third is *Waif* by Dallas Simpson, showing a little dark-

haired girl wearing a headscarf and ragged shawl. Its senti-
mental style is reflected in many other pictures of innocent
children, perhaps in tears and often with a small dog such as a
spaniel as their faithful companion.

All of these would, no doubt, be dismissed with some disgust
by art critics as bad art pandering to the masses. However, the
images obviously have a wide appeal. I think this may partly be
explained by their archetypal themes: a man and a woman in
love; the mysterious beauty from the Far East, a symbol of the
soul or the anima in Jungian terms; and the innocent child, an
archetypal symbol.

If, now, we turn to another triad of works of art – Rodin's
sculpture *The Kiss*, Botticelli's painting *The Birth of Venus* and
Picasso's painting *Child with a Dove* – we find just the same
themes addressed, though this time in works that would be
considered inspired by the same art critics. What it tells me is
that such archetypal images are indeed universal, common to
everyone whatever their social status, education, intelligence
quotient, or religious belief. There may be variations in the
sophistication with which they are expressed, but the essence
remains. And a beggar may even dream more richly than a king.

One man I visited lived in a halfway house close to his
hospital. He was alcoholic and had successfully stopped
drinking. I was asked to see him because he had an incurable
cancer of the throat brought on by his hard drinking. He shared
a large room with another inmate. The room was decorated with
cheap reproductions of dozens of famous paintings which he
had cut out of magazines and newspapers and stuck on the
walls. They cost him almost nothing but made a striking display.
A pile of dog-eared books on his bedside table was evidence of
his enjoyment of reading. Although he had the weather-beaten
look of a tramp, and bloodshot eyes, a legacy of his drinking, he
seemed to me very peaceful. I was touched by the way he had
created a life for himself, one which included the power of

images and of the written word. He knew and accepted that his cancer wasn't curable. He had friends among the others living in the same house. I felt that, despite his diagnosis, his soul had healed. Although he was still relatively well when I saw him, I wasn't surprised to hear that he died not long afterwards. He was ready to go.

A Holiday Dislocation

It was evening, shortly after the sun had set, and the light was fading as I parked our rental car, having dropped off my wife and children at our holiday apartment. We were having a beach holiday in Turkey. The cool of the evening was beginning to bring people out to stroll. I walked along the street past a block of flats on my right. A woman came out of the main door, obviously upset. Did I speak English? Yes. Did I know how to contact a doctor because her husband had hurt his shoulder?

Now this is a recurring dilemma for me, as for any doctor. If I see an accident, do I say I am a doctor and get involved – or not? My approach is to ask myself if my input is necessary. If it isn't, I walk away. If it is, so be it. So I told the woman I was a doctor and could I help? She looked at me gratefully and led me into her apartment. Her husband, Terry, was sitting on a sofa in the sitting room, wincing with pain and holding his right shoulder. His daughter, Annie, aged about seven, was sitting nearby, pale and wide-eyed as she looked silently at her father. Terry told me that he had had recurrent dislocations of his shoulder and he had put it out playing tennis. I examined him and it was obvious that he had indeed dislocated his shoulder again. I knew that relieving this might need treatment in hospital. However, I asked him to lie face down on his bed with the affected arm hanging down. Sometimes this allows a dislocation to reduce naturally. Then I went back to talk to his wife, Celia, and Annie in the sitting room.

I explained Terry might need to go to hospital and so it would be necessary to call a local doctor to arrange this. Annie burst into tears. She had been terrified at seeing her Dad ill and groaning in pain, and the prospect of hospital was even more frightening. It was easy to imagine how scary it must be to see one of the two main pillars of her life suddenly vulnerable and hurting. I could see that this had been traumatic for Annie; it had overwhelmed her coping mechanisms. Adults would be able to reason that such an injury could be dealt with successfully and would not be too concerned. Annie saw only that there was something very wrong with her Dad. I spent a long time trying to reassure her that her Dad would be OK. I only hope that this helped her, although I didn't then have the skills for working with traumatised children.

I helped Celia to find the phone number of an on-call doctor and said I would look in again to see how Terry was getting on since it would take some time before the doctor visited.

Half an hour later, I returned to find the dislocation had spontaneously reduced and a much relieved Terry sitting in an armchair with Celia, also much relieved, looking on and Annie calmer but still hypervigilant and wide-eyed, this the residue of her body's emergency reaction to what had happened. We talked for a while and I remember Terry was rather disappointed when I suggested that he avoid playing tennis for the rest of their holiday. It was as though he was already forgetting what had happened to him. Perhaps that was why he had had repeated dislocations.

For me, the lesson from this story is not so much Terry's injury, which is common enough, but the effect on his family, particularly Annie. Children can be traumatised by events that we adults would not imagine could have such an effect. And, since there are effective short-term therapies available, how important it is to recognise what is happening to the child as soon as possible and take action.

Chapter 7

Compassion

Compassion comes from the Latin *cum* meaning with, and *pati* meaning suffer; so, to suffer with. However, to this sense of being in sympathy with another person's affliction, we can add the accompanying impulse, even compulsion, to take action to relieve that ill person's distress.

I remember an example of compassion in action from when I was twelve. I was flying back from Belgium alone. Nowadays I would probably have a label attached to me and been escorted on and off the plane by one of the air hostesses. But back then there were no such luxuries and I was left to fend for myself. When I landed at Heathrow, I discovered that the connecting plane I was due to catch home had been cancelled. I didn't know what to do so, feeling somewhat scared, I went to the airline information desk and asked for help. The attendant there, a young woman, took pity on me. First she retrieved my baggage, a complicated process since it was meant to be in transit. Then she set about arranging a seat on a train from Paddington. Having done this she discovered that the airline was running a freight plane down to my destination. She managed to arrange a seat on the plane and forewarned the officials in the departure lounge. All this took, I would think, a couple of hours. I was so grateful to her. She played down my thanks, checked I was all right and walked off. Later, I walked out to the twin-engine plane, which looked rather like the plane at the end of the film *Casablanca*. I climbed the three steps up to the door, went in and sat down. I was accompanied by two air hostesses who were catching a lift home. It was night, a cloudless, starry night with no wind. We could see the lights of southern England spread out below us and the coast unfolding as we flew. It was a beautiful sight. The air was so still that the plane, like a buzzing hornet, seemed to be suspended motionless in the dark ether. As a shy twelve year old I didn't quite feel up to making conversation with two beautiful air hostesses, so I buried my nose in my book, looked out of the window from time to time and thought about the kindness of a stranger.

Natalie

I was told this story by Metropolitan Anthony Bloom, a Russian Orthodox archbishop; it was a story he also wrote about in one of his books. (1971, pp. 45–7) He described a poignant encounter in which a woman gave her life to save the lives of a mother and her children. It was 1919 and Russia was in the grip of a violent civil war. A woman, whose husband was an officer in the White Army, was trapped along with her two children and hiding in a cabin on the outskirts of a city taken by the Red Army. She planned to escape during a lull in the fighting. There was a knock at the door:

> She opened it in fear and was confronted by a young woman of her age. The woman (Natalie) said, "You must flee at once because you have been discovered and betrayed; you will be shot tonight." The other woman, showing her children who stood there, said, "How could we do that? We would be recognised at once, and they can't walk far." The young woman… said, "They won't look for you, I shall stay behind." And the mother said, "But they will kill you." "Yes," said the woman, "but I have no children, you must go." And the mother went… the cold of the early morning came and with it, death. The door was brutally opened and they did not take the trouble of dragging her out. She was shot where she was.

This was compassion taken to its ultimate point. Whenever I feel oppressed by the stories of violence and war that we see daily on our television screens, I remember stories such as this one and feel, not despair, but optimism. If we humans are capable of such altruism, there must be hope for us.

A Little Night Hitchhiking

Sometimes gifts are overwhelming in their unexpected generosity. I am thinking of a time when I was a medical student, and a friend and I were hitchhiking through France back to England. We were about 100 miles south of Paris. The sun had set and no one was stopping to give us a lift. We decided to walk about ten miles along a minor road to the beginning of a new motorway, sleep in a field overnight and then be up early next morning when we hoped drivers would be more likely to take pity on us.

As we walked along the dust on the edge of the road, darkness fell. Cars were infrequent and they were always announced by their brilliant yellow headlights; when they had passed us I would watch their shining red tail lights vanishing into the distance. Much of the time we were in the true, natural, dense darkness of the country. Above us the stars came out. The moon had not risen. We were hungry – we hadn't been able to buy any food for the evening – and weary from walking and fruitless hitchhiking. Nevertheless I was looking forward to sleeping under the stars.

A car passed us and then slowed down and stopped perhaps fifty yards ahead of us. It was open country so it could only have been for us. I felt uneasy. Who would stop at night to give two strangers a lift? Nevertheless, there were two of us and one of him so we hurried up to the car. The driver, in his twenties, asked if we needed a lift. Absolutely. We were heading north to Paris – as was he. Our lift said first that he had been driving back from Lyons and had been having some trouble with the brakes if we didn't mind. Not at all, I said, outwardly unfazed by this news. We needed the lift. Our host, Jean-Paul, turned out to be a psychologist who was returning to residential accommodation near Paris for students training in psychology.

There was a pause as he drove and he then hesitantly asked if we needed a place to stay overnight as there would be space in the hostel. My friend and I could hardly believe our luck. Two hours later, we turned into a short drive leading to the courtyard of a large building. Jean-Paul took us inside where there were a few students in the main hall. He took us to the kitchen, gave us supper and then showed us a two-bedded room, our accommodation for the night. Next morning, after breakfast, he said, apologetically, that he would offer to drive us to Paris but he didn't have money for the petrol. We agreed that we would pay. He drove us up to the outskirts of Paris and then took the *Peripherique*, the ring road around Paris, and dropped us off on a road heading north to Calais. We couldn't stop thanking him.

Looking back, I still find it hard to believe that one person would show so much kindness to two strangers and put himself to so much trouble on their behalf. I even sometimes wonder if it was a dream, it seemed so unlikely. Restoring one's faith in human nature – such an overused phrase. Nevertheless I do remember thinking that this stranger's generosity made me believe again in the essential goodness of the human heart.

Slowing Down

I was on an Intercity 125 train from London, Paddington, going down to the West Country, sitting in a window seat facing the direction of travel and no one opposite so I was able to stretch my legs out. A couple of books waited patiently to be read. Everything needed for a relaxing journey was to hand. Bliss. Trains are a great way of giving yourself permission to do nothing. As the train gathered speed, I found myself looking out of the window and idly speculating that, in principle, anything could happen at any time, that our best-laid plans can go adrift. Why I should have been thinking such thoughts I don't know, but a few minutes later, the train began to slow down from its 125 mph cruising speed and was soon travelling at about 20 mph. I assumed this was part of managing the many trains that travelled on this line. About five minutes later, a voice over the intercom asked for a doctor to come to the front of the train. I looked around. No one was getting up so either there were no other doctors around or, if there were, they were keeping quiet. I got up, walked the length of the train and identified myself to an agitated attendant. He said one of the drivers had taken ill and asked me to follow him through to the cabin at the front of the train. He opened the door from the carriage into the locomotive itself and I found myself edging along a caged walkway with the huge, roaring engine consisting, it seemed to me, chiefly of a deafening, giant, spinning flywheel, on my right. He opened another door and we walked through to the driver's cabin.

There were two drivers. The one on the left had slumped over sideways, while the one on the right had his hands tightly clenched over the controls, his eyes wide open with shock. He told me haltingly that the other, main, driver had suddenly lost consciousness and so he had taken over control of the train and slowed it down. It was at once obvious that the slumped driver had had a cardiac arrest. His pupils were widely dilated. This meant that his brain had been starved of oxygen for more than three minutes, which implied irreversible brain damage. I knew, too, that the time from slowing the train after he collapsed until I arrived was nearing ten minutes. There was no resuscitation equipment in the cabin. His chances of recovery were, effectively, nil.

My main concern, as soon as I had decided this, was to support the other driver. He was still shocked, so I took time to explain to him what had happened to his co-driver, I talked him through what he was planning – he was going to stop at the next station – and listened to him as he told me the story. I was really acting as an empathic, listening ear, giving him the attention he needed, while his adrenaline-soaked body gradually calmed. A part of me watched with fascination the empty line ahead – this was the first time I had ever had such a view. We pulled at last into Reading station, who, forewarned, had called an ambulance to take the collapsed driver to hospital. To my relief, British Rail provided another set of drivers. My cabin companion was in no state to continue. We helped get the driver off the train, on to a stretcher and into the ambulance. I got back into a carriage and walked slowly back to my seat. No one took any notice of me or of the crowd on the platform. It felt surreal as if two different worlds had been unfolding in parallel, unaware of each other. As I sat down, I thought, with sorrow, of the wife of the dead driver. I had been told he had had two previous heart attacks, but, even so, the news of her husband's death would still be unexpected and shocking to her.

It seemed ironic that a man with serious cardiac problems was driving a high-speed train. It felt like a shockingly apt metaphor for the way we force ourselves to work ever harder, even when we are unwell, to maintain our 125 mph pace of life. The cliche of the driven executive who considers himself indispensable and who dies of a heart attack at the age of 50, leaving a bereaved partner and young children, does sadly happen.

It's a question for all of us. Are we prepared to slow down? A difficult prescription, perhaps, but surely a better alternative to suicide by coronary artery occlusion or the many other ills we visit on ourselves.

The Battle of the Pillows

Formerly an independent woman, she had become very disabled by motor neurone disease. There was hardly any movement left in her limbs and her speech was markedly affected, with that characteristic slow, slurred, whining quality, interspersed with gulps of air, that people with this condition get. Not surprisingly, she was distressed by the effects of her illness on her. This became especially evident at bedtime. The hospice nurses would go into her room to fix her pillows for the night. This was a vital operation. She needed to be sitting at about 45° with pillows supporting her body so that it did not topple to one side, and further pillows to do the same for her head so that her breathing was not obstructed. Then there were her arms. They had to be just so – in other words in a comfortable position – and placed so that she could press her bell with the least movement of her fingers should some problem arise during the night. She was very fussy, understandably so since she was effectively completely helpless.

Sometimes this process would take an hour to get right. Over and over again, a certain pillow would be not quite as she wanted it – it needed to be a little more plump, or perhaps the opposite. The angle of her head was of prime importance and multiple adjustments needed to be made. If moving one pillow achieved the desired support, another pillow might have moved as a result and had to be readjusted. Sometimes I would walk past her room in the evening and see a couple of the nurses in their sky-blue uniforms patiently adjusting and readjusting the pillows in accordance with her slow instructions. I would see her lined, drawn and anxious face and chestnut brown hair, framed by her padded pillows, catch the pale gold of her angled wall lamp. I wondered at the extraordinary patience of the nurses.

It would be easy to speculate that there had been some event, some trauma in her past life that had spawned a psychological pattern of deep anxiety which had surfaced again in response to her illness. Perhaps so. Just as important, though, was the response of the nursing staff. They listened and they were prepared to take endless pains in getting it right for her. Their message could be summarised as: "We're here and we won't let you fall." For falling must have been one of her most profound fears: her head or body falling sideways, her arms slipping down the side of the bed out of reach of her bell – her lifeline – or, worst of all, her falling on to the floor. Children need the reassurance of their parents' arms to know that they will be held and not fall. So with her – and her unwelcome, enforced return to the helplessness of a newborn baby. No wonder she needed to stay in control of her pillows.

What the nurses were doing would never make headline news. There was none of the drama or kudos associated with famous clinical advances such as the discovery of penicillin. What they were doing was not for the whole world, but just for that individual at one particular time. Yet what they provided was of the greatest importance to one ill woman frightened of dying. It was an act of compassion on their part, of recognising the humanity of another person and responding from their own humanity. I call that worthwhile.

Chapter 8

Hope

On 10th May 1940, Belgium, though following a policy of neutrality after the outbreak of the Second World War, was invaded by German armed forces and 18 days later it was under an occupation which was to last till September 1944. My mother and grandparents were living in Ghent at this time. They experienced not only the humiliation of being ruled by a German military government, but also the realities of life under occupation: strict rationing of food, fuel and clothing, the black market, collaboration, forced labour, deportation of Belgian Jews to the concentration camps and Allied bombing raids which killed civilians. I wonder what it was like to walk down familiar streets and see the German flag with its swastika flying over public buildings and to walk past German soldiers who might stop you and check your papers at any time. My mother didn't talk much about it and I wonder now how they kept going, kept hope alive.

It was when she talked about food that I got a different perspective. Rationing meant that everyone was hungry so food became of consuming interest, so to speak. Like many others, she used to ride out on her bike to country farms belonging to friends or family. Though much of the produce of the farms was commandeered by the Germans, there would still be enough for her to take back a package hidden under her skirts. She had to pass German checkpoints on the way back; if she had been caught, she would have faced a punitive fine and detention. Here was a spirit of opposition, I thought, a small subversion of the hated regime. What it must have been like when Ghent was liberated and their hopes of freedom fulfilled, I can only imagine.

Hope and healing go together, but not, perhaps, in the way that you might think. Hope is crucial; it's what drives us through life, like the wind making sails belly out. It is a lifelong way of being. It's a choice. It keeps you going when times are bad, when it seems nothing is right, when you wish life would flow, but, obstinately, it doesn't. With hope, goes hard, hard work, years of inner effort and tiny day-to-day alterations that are nigh on imperceptible. You have a feeling that nothing is changing and nothing ever will. But step back, turn around and look over your life, the last year, the last decade even, and suddenly, surprised, you will see a difference. One stick is nothing, weak, easily broken. A bundle of sticks gathered over time is strong and cannot be snapped.

So, yes, we need hope for healing, and we need application, practising over and over again an attitude of trust. One day we can't get life at all and, the next, something shifts inside and we have moved forward, we understand, we re-member who we always were, we accept.

Hope is also about tenacity, holding on, gritting your teeth, not sliding into a soft, grey, passive slump of anergy. It's like your dog holding fast to one end of a stick and you the other. you're playing but his teeth are bared and you can hear the low growls in his throat and his fierce determination. So we need to keep hoping, for it's a primer for health. You can be ill or even dying and still live in a whole – wholistic – way whatever the contingencies and restrictions of your physical being. Imagine what it would be like to keep your mind, your very soul focused on your true hope, the purpose of your life. Think of the people who have done that. Helen Keller became deaf and blind following an illness when she was two years old. Despite this, she learned to read, write and speak, and was awarded a degree. She was a political activist, and became world famous as a lecturer and author. Nelson Mandela (1995) had to contend with imprisonment for nearly 28 years – it would have been so very easy to give up. "I have a dream," said Martin Luther King as he faced down the menace of racism in the Southern United States. What they have in common is their inner strength and their determination to live the life they were born for. Mount Sinai in Egypt is sacred to Judaism, Christianity and Islam. Mount Kailash in Tibet is sacred to Buddhists, Hindus, Jains and Böns. Uluru in Australia is sacred to Aborigines. Mount Shasta in California is sacred to Native Americans. In so many religious traditions, mountains are metaphors for self-realisation, and hermits, ascetics, holy men and the like tell us that there are a thousand paths, not one set way, that lead to the summit. It is for each person to find their own path. And we get lost, we follow tracks that lead nowhere, we face unclimbable cliffs, we hide from predators, we fall, we are injured, we are at the mercy of storms, mists and snows.

But when we arrive at last and join the others that have reached this same summit, we can look down and see the whole path we have trodden and be amazed that we have come so far, have overcome such obstacles. It is the journey of a lifetime.

But what of those who have fallen into despair, who have lost hope, who no longer wish to try to live? How are we to help? It is hard for us just to be with someone who feels this way. We want to find something, anything that will relieve their pain (and our discomfort). We try, to use an analogy from quantum mechanics, to collapse the wave function of many possibilities into just one: "We'll try another cycle of chemotherapy." Or: "We could enter you into our research trial." Or: "You must think positive." Or: "Let's get you a ticket to Switzerland to that clinic that does assisted suicides." Or: "Smile, Jesus loves you." Or: "I'll just get you a sedative." Or: "don't talk like that; I can't stand it." And so on.

Imagine a man. It is night and very cold. He is lying sprawled on the ground. Around him are ancient, twisted, Arthur

Rackham olive trees. He is in the grip of terror. Drops of cold sweat fall from his pallid face and track through his hair. His heart is thumping fast and hard like a drum. He trembles, but not from cold. He knows what is going to happen: arrest, torture, execution. He has asked his friends to watch with him. They are a little way away, asleep. He wakes them with the same request; soon they fall asleep again. He is alone with his anguish.

It would be hubris, I think, to imagine that we can know the right answer when another human being faces despair. True, we can offer ideas but these may or may not be accepted. Perhaps most important is that phrase, one of Dame Cicely Saunders' favourites, "Watch with Me", the request Jesus made – without success – to his disciples in the Garden of Gethsemane. When all else has gone, there remains the simple presence of one person to another who, even if he has lost hope, knows he is not alone.

The Importance of Being Scottie

As a child, I was very fond of a glove puppet I had whose name was Scottie, since he was a Scottish terrier. He became very battered over time. One glass eye had a squint, which endeared me to him, since I had the same. I used to try rotating his eye to correct the squint but, somehow, it always slipped back into its former position. His artificial fur was black and he had two very upright ears and grey whiskers. The right whisker was a bit wild so I tried snipping it back. Unfortunately, I over-snipped and he was left with one short and one long moustache. I wasn't bothered. He was fine just as he was.

For a while, Scottie was my constant companion. Putting him on meant my index finger went into the short papier mâché tunnel inside his head, while my third finger was his left arm and my thumb was his right arm. This made for a marked and pleasing unevenness in his upper limb dexterity – on the left was skill and fine movements, on the right, no-nonsense brawn. He even came cycling with me. He held the left handlebar while I held the right – it seemed a fair division of labour.

The thing I liked most about him was that he was a wonderful listener. If I was upset about anything or lonely, he was the best confidant I could wish for. He would look at me quietly, giving me his complete attention. I could tell him anything. Somehow, I knew he might not have the answers I was looking for, but that didn't matter. He listened. He never judged me. He understood.

No doubt Scottie was a form of transitional object. No doubt, too, I projected my own need for listening and understanding on to him. For me, though, whatever the analytic reasoning, our partnership was a great success. Scottie helped me through difficult times.

Anyone who has visited a children's ward in hospital or a

children's hospice could not fail to see the crowds of toys, dolls, teddy bears and the like. These are important objects for the sick children. They represent something real and significant in their inner world and need to be respected as such. They can be seen as an aspect of each child's soul writ large. We may not know what; they may not want to let us into their secret. However, making sure that the ever-faithful Teddy accompanies a child to her operation, or that Bunny, the trusted confidant, is on hand to be tucked in at night with his owner, are important ways of helping children to feel safe. It is no wonder that the story of the *Velveteen Rabbit* (Williams 2004), who is loved so much that he becomes Real, is so cherished, and it is no wonder that so many children's stories start with toys in the playroom magically coming alive at night, maybe on the stroke of midnight. We adults instinctively know this, since we were children too. I remember when I used to read such bedtime stories to my children, it was no chore, I enjoyed them as much as they did.

The Safe Place

Finding safety is a basic animal – and human – instinct. It is so fundamental to how we live that we don't even notice it; but look around and you'll see it everywhere in action. Watch children in a playground and safety is played out in any number of ways. Here is a three year old who has fallen and grazed his knee. His mother quickly picks him up and hugs him, and kisses the sore place better; his tears soon subside. There is another mother holding her toddler who is at the top of a slide. Cautiously, the mother starts her daughter sliding slowly downwards, holding on all the time; the little girl loves it. Nearby a mother is rescuing her son from an older boy who is trying to steal his yellow plastic atomic ray gun. A five year old is hanging upside down from a climbing frame, swinging back and forth. Her aunt calls out a warning. Yes, safety and how much we feel able to take risks are part of the fabric of our lives.

People with cancer are often traumatised by their illness or their treatment, as are for that matter those close to them. When their fear is running out of control, I sometimes suggest a meditation called 'the safe place' to them. I ask them to close their eyes and visualise a place in nature, either somewhere real or imagined, a place where they feel totally safe. I ask them to look around and see what they see in as much detail as possible – perhaps a forest or the sea, a lake or a mountain. Then we slowly go through each of the other senses – hearing, touch, smell, movement – in the same way. Lastly, I ask them to mentally touch something – bark or rock or sand – to act as a sensory reminder, a mental anchor.

How does this work in practice? Imagine a woman, let's call her Sarah. Just an ordinary person, like any other. She discovers she has cancer of the colon. It's treatable says her doctor briskly, and so she submits herself to surgery and radiotherapy. And all this time the tightness that has seized her throat, bound her chest so that she can scarcely breathe and knotted her stomach, stays with her. A good chance that you're cured, she's told at the end of her treatment. So, why am I so depressed, she wonders a month later. In therapy her shock state begins to unfreeze and she discovers her feelings about her cancer for the first time; panic overwhelms her. That night, she sleeps and dreams again of the time her older stepbrother raped her when she was seven. She wakes, sweating, shaking and sobbing. As she talks to her therapist, the memory of her terror returns. Imagine a place of safety, she is told, I'll guide you through it. So she does. And gradually her fear subsides, her pulse slows, her breathing calms. You can return here any time, she is reminded. Back home, she writes it down. It might go something like this:

… I yearn for something more. A secret place, spacious and quiet. I see a pool, utterly transparent with a faint, bluish bloom from the sun's rays which sparkle on the surface when a faint wind catches the skin of the water like a cat's paw. I can feel the wind, soft on my skin and smell the mountain flowers. Somewhere nearby, a curlew calls, a melodious riff. There is a curving bluish-grey granite outcrop across the pool. I dive into the cool, translucent water and follow the rock face down and down and find pebbles and sand glittering in the light at the bottom. A fish with blue, grey and gold scales and thick rubbery lips glides calmly past me in iridescent splendour. My head breaks the water's surface and a thousand drops fall in curtains from my hair, brilliant jewels, while ever-widening ripples spread across the pool. I taste the cold, clean water…

As she writes, she experiences once again the calmness she felt earlier. When she goes to bed she feels a little more confidence. Should her nightmare return, she is no longer helpless.

This is a simple meditation and yet I am repeatedly surprised at how effective it is. It is like watching a storm blow over or the sun come out from behind dark clouds. Best of all, the feared emotional pain is eased, something traumatised people long for. This is also a resource that is open to us all since each of us will have our own store of healing memories to draw on.

'Soul' comes from two roots: the Greek word, *aiolos*, meaning coloured, mobile, iridescent; and the Slavonic word, *sila*, meaning strength. Soul, then, "is a moving force, that is, life-force." (Jung, 1984, p. 209) By using imagery such as that described above, we strengthen the wavering life force of the traumatised soul.

Candles in the Window

It was a cold December night as Joan and I, carrying our newborn daughter, walked along the road to St Christopher's Hospice. Under the light of the stars we could see that the hospice was plunged in darkness. However, along every windowsill – and the front of St Christopher's is five storeys mostly made up of windows – were row upon row of glass jars with lit candles in them. It was an enchanting sight. We had come for the carols and tradition had it that a mother and newborn baby were to lead the procession, representing, of course, Mary and the infant Jesus. This year, it was our turn. We joined the other singers in the entrance foyer.

There was much rustling of carol sheets and testing of torches – for the wards would be in darkness. Joan was called by Dame Cicely Saunders to the head of the procession. They made a strange pair; Dame Cicely was about nine inches taller than her. Luckily our baby was asleep having been bribed with a large slug of breast milk shortly before. I, a modern day Joseph I suppose, took my humble place among the other singers.

We set off and entered the first ward, singing as we went. The ward consisted of a corridor off which were open-plan four-bedded bays. Our carolling crocodile wove slowly around the beds. In the dim light of the candles we could see each patient in bed with their family sitting with them. If a patient was alone, one of the nurses sat with him. No one was left alone. The atmosphere was magical, tender and soulful. Slowly we made our way through each of the other three wards, watched by the patients' shining eyes reflected in the candlelight. Everyone, singers and watchers alike, was moved by the occasion. This was something shared; all were equal participants.

There was more. As we walked, we moved, as it were, through an invisible cloud of memories – memories of the tens of thousands of patients and their loved ones who had occupied these beds over the years. We were remembering them through this ritual.

Up ahead, Joan was being given commanding *sotto voce* instructions by Dame Cicely, who liked things just so – "Stop!" "Start walking again!" "Slow down!" Fortunately, our newborn remained blissed out on her milk and took no notice of events around her.

The candle in the window is an old Polish tradition. It is lit on Christmas Eve to welcome the Christ child. At the same time an extra place is laid at the table in case a traveller should pass by looking for a place to stay, as did Joseph searching from house to house for lodgings in Bethlehem.

It seems strange that this story about the beginning of a life should be re-enacted in song in a hospice, a place where people are coming to the end of their lives. Yet there are similarities. Both are about a life transition; indeed nurses caring for the dying are sometimes called midwives. In both there is the theme of journeying and the search for a place to stay, a place of refuge, whether this be a stable or a hospice. The child is central to both, whether this be the Christ child or the inner child that we all have within us, a child that may be deeply distressed and in need of comfort. The name Christopher means Christ-bearer harking back to the story of St Christopher, known for his great strength, who on a wild night carried the Christ child across a raging river, the heaviest burden he had ever had to bear; an apt name for a hospice then.

And this was a healing ritual. It wasn't the stated intention, but it certainly had that effect. For myself, I found the tensions of the day dissolving gradually as we made our rounds. I could feel shivers down my spine, a response to the beauty and pathos of the moment. I sensed we were on a different plane of reality for a little while. Maybe this is how healing often works. Rather than a spectacular miracle there is a simple and subtle shift towards wholeness that comes upon us unbidden and sometimes unnoticed. It works both ways, too, not only for the sick but for those who care for them.

Bulba!

My chief memory of Aurelia is of her writing. She had been admitted to my hospice with motor neurone disease since she could no longer cope at home. She looked somewhat like a benign witch with long, straggly, black hair, dark eyes and a curved nose. While her arms and legs were still partly functional, her swallowing and speech had been badly affected. This meant that she needed help with eating a special soft diet, and that she could only communicate by nods and gestures and by writing. Hers, however, was no ordinary writing. She would seize her pen and paper and scrawl her looping, untidy script at high speed, her arm moving in synchrony as if conducting an orchestra playing an energetic piece. Not for her neat, tidy little letters that followed prescriptive lines. No. Her writing was big and bold. Line after line would be penned, sheets of paper covered and discarded in drifts on her bed. She was a communicator, and if she couldn't speak, she could at least write. Conversations with her were never boring.

In a way, her writing was her lifeline, her way of maintaining some control over her paralysing illness. However, even before she became ill, words had been important to her. She was an author and poet, and she wrote sonnets to her illness, which she christened Bulba. There was a reason for this. The area of the brain that controls the motor commands to swallow or speak is called the bulbar region, and Aurelia's affliction was accordingly a bulbar palsy. She had given her illness a personality and a name which might have come from Greek mythology. A phrase in one of her poems went thus: "by Bulba overcome." For some reason this has stuck in my memory, partly perhaps because I never saw a person less overcome by her illness than Aurelia.

She was an ardent spiritualist, as was a good friend of hers who visited her every day. They had 'conversations', spoken and written, about when it would be her time to cross over and how they would meet again in the next life. Aurelia knew perfectly well that she would die soon and she faced her illness head on. Most people, however courageously they confront their impending death, will have times of feeling frightened and tearful. If Aurelia did, it wasn't obvious – and I knew she wasn't pretending. Death for her wasn't frightening. She was serious about her beliefs and she was ready to pass over when her time came, and I think looked forward to it.

I recall seeing her face after she had died. She had the look of a warrior in repose. That phrase about fighting the good fight seemed to fit her well. And now, even after all these years, I still see her in my mind's eye energetically conducting her orchestra of words in a *finale furioso*.

Chapter 9

Truth

There are some lines from Shakespeare that have kept coming back to me over the years. They are from Hamlet. Polonius is speaking to Laertes:

This above all: to thine own self be true,
And it must follow, as the night the day,
Thou canst not then be false to any man.
(Shakespeare: *Hamlet*. 1:3:79–80)

How many of us are really true to our own self? The story of Byron Katie (Katie 2002, pp. *xi–xii*) speaks to this. She was a real estate manager in California and experienced a ten-year fall into profound depression, rage, paranoia and despair. At one stage she decided to check into a halfway house for women with eating disorders. One morning she woke up – she had been sleeping on the floor – and found she had no concept of who or what she was:

There was no me… All my rage, all the thoughts that had been troubling me, my whole world, the whole world, was gone. At the same time, laughter welled up from the depths and just poured out. Everything was unrecognizable. It was as if something else had woken up. It opened its eyes. It was looking through Katie's eyes. And it was so delighted. It was intoxicated with joy. There was nothing separate, nothing unacceptable to it; everything was its very own self.

She had, I think, discovered what Buddhists call our true nature. She has described this as being like coming across a rattlesnake in the desert, experiencing terror and then realising with profound relief it is just a piece of rope. (Katie 2005, pp. *xvii–xviii*) When she returned home, she was transformed. Her intense psychological distress had disappeared, her formerly angry relationship with her children healed and people would spontaneously come and talk to her, looking for help.

It takes a lot for us to let fall our defensive barriers, those ramparts carefully set up to hide what we consider to be our faults from others. And this falling apart is just what crises do, as I discovered repeatedly whenever I worked medically with people in emergency situations. They would be open, their walls had come down, they were real. Too ill to protest, they had to trust the medical and nursing team. They were naked physically, emotionally and spiritually. It was a privilege, an intimacy, to be allowed to see people in this state. The strange thing was this: a few days later when they felt better their defences might well have sprung up again and there would be a polite distance between us. It seems it is hard to remain open for long.

Some years ago, I came across a wonderfully vivid comment on this by the Buddhist nun Pema Chödrön in her book, *When Things Fall Apart* (1997, p. 118):

The truth, said an ancient Chinese Master, is neither like this nor like that. It is like a dog yearning over a bowl of burning oil. He can't leave it, because it is too desirable, and he can't lick it because it is too hot.

Perhaps it is when we face death that we are most likely to discover our true nature. This was most movingly demonstrated in the 9/11 disaster in New York in 2001. Knowing they were about to die, people on the planes on collision course with the World Trade Center phoned their loved ones. Flight attendant Ceecee Lyles left a message for her husband: "Please tell my children that I love them very much. I'm sorry, baby. I wish I could see your face again." Elizabeth Rivas' husband phoned his young daughter from the World Trade Center; she reported: "He say, mommy, he say he love you no matter what happens, he loves you." Others said: "Tell Billy I never stopped loving him and forgave him long ago," and "Pray for me, Father. Pray for me, I haven't been very good." Captain Walter Hynes one of the firemen who died in the disaster left a message for his family: "I don't know if we'll make it out. I want to tell you that I love you and I love the kids." There is no record of any grievances being aired nor, and this is extraordinary, of any condemnation of the terrorists. (Noonan 2006) It seems, then, that when everything else has been stripped away, we find that love is our true nature.

Enough Is Enough

I feel sad when I remember Winifred and yet she taught me so much even if she didn't know it. She was an elderly lady, tall and round-shouldered, grey haired and with an animated expression as she talked. She had been admitted for investigation of gastric symptoms. She was found to have a cancer at the junction between her stomach and oesophagus. Curative surgery was indicated and I went to see her to obtain her consent. We went through what the surgery entailed, and the risks, including what is, in dry medical parlance, called operative mortality, known to be higher in the elderly. She thought for a while and then said: "It's a big one... but I think I'll do it," as though she were embarking on an exciting, risky adventure. She took the pen and signed the consent form.

Her Christian faith was very important to her, and an elderly couple from her church came to visit her most days since she had no close relatives living.

I don't remember anything untoward happening during her long operation. Afterwards, Winifred slowly regained consciousness and was taken back to her ward. Over the next few days we monitored her closely, but, somehow, she did not pick up and recover. She slept much of the time. She was weak and had no energy. She felt unwell. There was nothing specific to explain her lack of progress. The days turned into a week, then two weeks, and if anything she grew worse. Weeks passed and she became intermittently confused.

Every morning, I would cross the old Victorian hospital courtyard, with its stone paving flags, enter the ward through its scuffed, wooden, glass-panelled swing doors, walk across the noisy parquet flooring to the sister's desk and get a report from the nurse in charge. It was the same every day. Winifred was no better. I felt frustrated that there was nothing I could do and guilty as if I were failing in some way. Every day, too, we would check her abdominal wound. It refused to heal even after weeks had passed and she had gone back to the operating theatre for re-suturing. In hindsight, nothing could have been clearer. Her body's message was that it had passed the stage of healing.

I talked one day with Winifred's friends who continued to visit her faithfully. They gently suggested that it didn't look as though she was going to get better. I disagreed. I felt we should keep trying.

A week or so later, I was on call, and was asked to see Winifred since her condition has suddenly worsened. Yet again I crossed the courtyard, at night this time. Yet again my feet clacked across the parquet floor. She was now in a side-room. She was semiconscious, her breathing fast and rattling, her skin grey. A chest X-ray confirmed she had bronchopneumonia. Still in my driven, active mode, I set up a drip and started her on intravenous antibiotics. Slowly, over the next few days, her pneumonia improved. However, she didn't. She remained very frail, and, little by little, her condition again worsened.

This was the point at which I gave up trying to get her better. In a haze of secret shame, I watched, helpless, as she slid towards death, which mercifully took her some days later. Her friends continued to visit and sit with her. Their support was of much greater value to her during this time than my doomed attempts at heroic medicine.

Variations on this story still happen in hospitals around the world. True, medical technology is now much more advanced than when Winifred was treated, 35 years ago. Nevertheless, the question remains the same. When is it time to stop? Generation after generation of newly qualified doctors have struggled with this issue.

Winifred's story was a lesson for me. Trying to keep someone such as her alive causes unnecessary suffering and changes the process of dying from a natural event to a long drawn-out distressing struggle, distressing not only for the patient but for their loved ones too. People are not just machines to be put right. There is indeed a time to die. To deny this is medical hubris.

I was also discovering how limited medicine is, despite the extraordinary advances in health care of the last century. The neat formulations of diagnosis and treatment set out in medical textbooks so often fall short in the real world. People frequently have illnesses that do not seem to fit any diagnostic category. Others have the correct treatment for their condition but, like Winifred, they just don't get better.

My abiding memory is of Winifred's friends. They might be called nondescript to outward appearances. The strange thing is that, although I have only a partial memory of what they looked like physically, their presence remains with me, as though they were bigger on the inside than the outside. They kept faith with her.

A Dark Horse

During childhood holidays by the beach in Belgium, my parents would sometimes take me, my brother and my sister riding on the sands. This, however, was no stroll on a donkey. As we walked along the beach towards our equine rendezvous, we would see, in the distance, a group of tethered horses waiting patiently for riders. The horses' owner was called Eugene. He was a retired jockey, small, wiry and spare with pale blue eyes, fair hair and a tanned, weathered face. He always wore a cloth cap, riding boots and jodhpurs. He would bring the horses over from his stables a mile or so away inland and wait for customers. Once he had gathered a quorum, he would lead us all along the hard wet sand, past breakwaters which lined the beach for miles either way. Walking and trotting were the usual modes and I gradually learned how to sit up and then down rhythmically to stop bucketing around when we were trotting. Cantering was a dream of the future. Returning, we would follow the line of hoof prints made on the way out. Every now and then, one of the horses deposited an offering of dung on the sand; it sat there patiently, waiting to be swept away by the next tide.

The horses were a varied lot. Some were like ponies drawn by the cartoonist, Thelwell – short, stout and wide in the back, which meant one had to stick one's legs out sideways – quite uncomfortable. Riding them was a bit like riding on a bicycle over cobbles. At the other end of this equine gathering was a very tall horse – I think he had been a racehorse – a thoroughbred, long-legged and graceful. His coat was between darkest-brown and black, and shone in the sun. He had a white blaze on his forehead and was called *Satan*.[4] I was in awe of this superhorse – I was, after all, only nine years old at the time. His name suggested a dark, frightening past and I kept my distance from him. In between these two extremes were a mixed bag of brown horses of different hues and sizes, and one Palomino pony who I rather liked as he reminded me of stories from the Wild West. The Indians always rode Palominos, or so it seemed to me, and I could imagine myself in buckskin and long hair riding bareback across the plains where vast throngs of bison grazed, just waiting to be felled by my deadly arrows.

One day, Eugene decided I was ready to try cantering. He held the horse I was riding on a long lead and then with a few flicks of his whip – which didn't make contact – and a kind of kissing noise, he had my steed starting to walk, then trot and finally canter in a big circle following its own hoof prints in the sand till a churned-up ring had been formed on the beach. My heart beat fast as we moved into third gear but I loved the ease of cantering after the jerkiness of trotting, and felt exultant when I slid off my horse at the end of the session.

My last memory is of Eugene telling me one day I could ride on *Satan*. I felt a mixture of anxiety and excitement. I imagined *Satan* living up to his name and bolting or bucking me off. I had to be helped up into the saddle and the ground seemed a long way down. When we started, I realised my preconceptions about him were all wrong. My sense of his character, as we trekked across the sands, was not of some malign monster but actually a horse who was alert, friendly and easy to ride. I could tell he enjoyed these outings and was curious about what was going on around him. I was amazed at how smooth his movements were. He was a Rolls-Royce in comparison with the smaller horses that were more like Citroen 2CVs. His stride was so long I had to keep reining him in to keep pace with the others.

We often equate darkness with evil, death, destruction and hell. My horse was saddled with a name that implied this connection. In reality it was so inappropriate. And we also miss experiencing darkness as beautiful.

I am standing, along with several hundred other people, in

darkness and silence. A light flickers briefly ahead of us and flames rise from a brazier. Several men and children are grouped around the flames. Their faces glow red-gold in the light. One of the men, in gold and ivory vestments, takes a candle, four feet high, lights it from the brazier, and places it on a stand. Two children in white robes light tapers from it and turn to us, who each hold a small candle. They light the candles of those at the front, who in turn light those around them in a chain reaction. A slow wave of light spreads out and softly illuminates the church. Around the world the same ceremony of light is being performed following the sweep of night's shadow as it circles the globe.

I always find this Easter vigil ritual moving. While this is a service of the dawn of light, an essential part of it is the pregnant darkness in which illumination is born. Every living thing on the surface of our planet is attuned to this rhythm of darkness giving birth to light.

The end of life is often seen as a time of darkness, of suffering. Perhaps it can be friendly as well. I recall many whose faces changed as they approached their life-ending – and after. The lines of distress were smoothed away, the braced muscles relaxed; they looked years younger – and peaceful.

One of the laws of physics states that matter cannot be created or destroyed. It can only be converted to a different form, whether this be material or energetic. I think life is like that, too. It can't be destroyed but it can be transformed.

Vision Quests

If I think back over the times I have sat with patients and talked to them, there were a number of themes that kept recurring. There was loneliness. It didn't matter if the patient was surrounded by loved ones, still that sense of being utterly alone stayed with them. They were, after all, facing the prospect of death. Those about them could accompany them to the door, but the patient had to go through it alone. Then they might be faced with questions about their very existence: "What has been my purpose in living?" "Have I lived according to my values?" Thirdly, they might experience sights and sounds that others do not see or hear. They might see members of their family who have already died, for example. Usually these experiences are labelled as hallucinations or delusions by their carers. Fourthly, due to their advancing illness they may be able to eat or drink little or nothing.

Perhaps these apparently unconnected states have more in common than we might think. A traditional ritual from Native American cultures may cast some light on this. When a member of a tribe has an important question to consider, their medicine person may send him out into the wilderness with particular instructions – to go to a certain mountain or hilltop and sit there for a specified length of time, maybe several days, and observe what happens. They may be told to fast during this time, no food, no water. They then report back on whatever they experience, whether humble or dramatic, and their medicine person inter- prets it with respect to their question. Some will see visions, some might notice unusual behaviour in an animal, some might find their attention drawn to something seemingly insignificant such as patterns in the bark of a tree or the movement of grass. This is a vision quest, and it has the same four elements of aloneness, questioning, fasting and visions described above for the dying.

The time of dying may, then, not just be a random dissolution, but may also be seen as a quest, the last of many quests, great and small in a life, a quest that encompasses all the others.

There is a further aspect to this. The theme of searching runs through the world religions, as well as through mythological stories worldwide. In the West, the story of Jesus and his time in the wilderness is well known. Following his baptism, he was driven by the Spirit into the desert wilderness of Judaea. There he fasted and was with the wild animals as he wandered alone through the scarred, bleak and inhospitable landscape and was burned by the sun. There, too, he met his adversary, Satan, who tempted him through wild visions of power, of flying and of transforming matter. When he came back from this life-changing ordeal, the man who was an unknown carpenter was transformed. The people of his village could scarcely recognise him.

In the same way, the Buddha, in search of the truth, vowed to sit in meditation under a Bodhi tree until he had realised his aim. Legend has embroidered this simple story: enter the dread demon, Mara, who visited the Buddha with temptations. He sent armies of demons to attack him, but these dissipated when the Buddha simply touched the earth. Mara sent his three beautiful daughters to seduce the Buddha, but without success. As the demon and his forces retreated in confusion, the Buddha attained enlightenment; tradition has it that he had been meditating for 49 days.

Each person searches for their truth in their own way, whether this be dramatic as in the stories of Jesus and the Buddha, or quiet and hidden. Often the latter pertains for the dying, who may be very weak, unable to speak and increasingly drowsy. Nevertheless, their journeys through their unknown inner landscapes, veiled from the eyes of observers, may be of the utmost significance and, if this is an appropriate phrase for those close to death, life-changing.

Pain as a Gift

Chronic pain in long-term or end-stage illnesses may cause much suffering and treatment is rightly geared towards its suppression. There is, however, one chronic and much feared condition where the *absence* of pain contributes to the damage caused by the illness. A memory from childhood comes to mind. I was running across a landing barefoot. I stepped on a drawing pin I hadn't seen. My leg reacted, seemingly of its own volition. My knee flexed sharply lifting my foot away from the drawing pin even as I felt the sharp pain. Hopping on my other foot and wincing with the pain, I sat on the floor and lifted my foot up to remove the offending pin. I saw that it had only penetrated about two or three millimetres. My automatic self-protective withdrawal response had been that quick.

Usually we think of pain negatively. But its primary and vital function is to protect us from injury, as in my case, or in warning us of illness. Indeed, without pain we would be in serious trouble. This was brought home to me when, as a house surgeon, I looked after a man with Hansen's disease, or leprosy. He had been treated for many years and was no longer infectious but he had been left with the after-effects of his illness. He had lost some of his fingers and toes, he had to wear special boots with which to walk and the bridge of his nose was sunken. He was a lascar and had worked as a seaman on merchant ships sailing between Europe and India for many years. The surgical ward then was an old Nightingale ward – the hospital had been built in the 19th century – with rows of beds down each side. He would always call out a greeting as I made my way slowly along the ward, seeing each patient in turn. A cheerful man despite his condition, he was well used to hospitals – indeed he might have been called a professional patient – having been admitted for dozens of operations.

What had caused the damage? It used to be thought that it was the leprosy bacterium itself, causing so-called 'bad flesh'. Then a surgeon, Paul Brand (Yancey & Brand 1997), working in a missionary hospital in India, demonstrated that it was because the bacterium had invaded nerves carrying sensory signals from the extremities, which led to skin numbness in the hands and feet. Those affected could not feel anything if, for example, they picked up a hot metal saucepan, even if it caused their skin to blister; or if they picked up a piece of wood with a projecting nail, they would not notice that it had caused a wound. Indeed, Paul Brand found that if he shook hands with people with Hansen's disease, his hand would be almost crushed because they had no feedback sensory signals telling them to lighten their grip. Dr Brand saw how disastrous it was to have no pain sensation. It made him feel deeply grateful for this remarkable protective mechanism.

Being

Our cabin, sheltered by a grove of coconut trees, looked out on to the beach and the small bay beyond. It was the dry season and mosquito numbers were down. From our veranda, we could watch piratical, black frigate birds stealing fish from other birds, portly brown pelicans gliding low over the shining water in a V-shaped formation, laughing gulls laughing as they hung around the fishing boats and tiny, graceful yellow-billed terns hovering and diving whenever they glimpsed a fish just below the water's surface. To our right was a small village encircling the bay. The fishermen would go out early in the morning, their traditional brightly-painted wooden boats driven by powerful outboard motors. They would return before lunchtime and lay out their catches on stone slabs close to the beach, waiting for buyers. Kingfish, blackjack, bonita and streamlined, silvery tuna, some three or four feet in length.

We, meanwhile, would snorkel in the calm, clear waters of the bay and watch the fishes changing colour as they drifted through the multicoloured coral forests; occasionally we even saw a small turtle. Evenings, we could walk along to the pier and watch the sunset, oranges and golds fading to violet and then deep blue, which silhouetted the fishing boats against the reflected colours in the calm water.

There were very few tourists and the beach in front of our cabin was mostly used as a pathway by the villagers. Every now and then, one would stop and chat to us. You couldn't hurry in that sort of heat. One of them was called, of all things, Donald Duck, and he seemed to have all the time in the world. He would sometimes steal coconuts or fruit from his neighbours – it was the season for mangoes – and then sell them on to us. One day, my daughter asked him: "What do you do all day?" He thought for a moment. He talked first about how he went fishing. Then he said:

"But sometimes, ah does jus' be."

Now Donald was no saint, but somehow he seemed to have spontaneously discovered a way of life that saints have extolled and that seekers after the truth have struggled to realise for decades of their life. The incongruity made me laugh. I once came across another reminder in the same vein. It was an epitaph on a tombstone in Boothill Cemetery in Tombstone, Arizona: "Be what you is," it said, "cuz if you be what you ain't, then you ain't what you is." (Campbell 1990, p. xxiv) What was the story behind that sentence, I wondered? Who was the person who had decided it summed up his life so well he would put it on his gravestone?

Beingness, then, is not a task to be achieved like building a house, but rather a state, an essence, that has always been there within us, waiting to be uncovered. Buried treasure. The pearl of great price. Serious or life-threatening illnesses and the sense of vulnerability they engender may act as a catalyst to discovering being.

Real

I always liked the story of Pinocchio, the wooden puppet who wanted to become a real boy. I remember going to see the Walt Disney cartoon as a child. I recall especially the scene where he rescues Geppetto, his father, from the belly of Monstro the whale, only to be pursued by the enraged leviathan. Pinocchio swims the drowning Geppetto safely to shore, but is drowned himself in the tidal wave caused by the whale crashing into a cliff. I was in tears by this stage and welcomed with relief the Blue Fairy bringing Pinocchio back to life as a real flesh-and-blood boy at the end of the film.

This is, of course, an allegory about becoming alive, about being who we really are. Illness may facilitate – albeit as an unwelcome guest – this journey towards becoming real.

Joanne had contracted motor neurone disease, a condition that caused a gradual loss of strength in her limbs along with diffi-culties with swallowing and speaking. People with motor neurone disease are often uncannily similar in the way they struggle to speak or to swallow, almost as if they are related to each other.

Joanne had her home in one of the four-bedded bays of a hospice where I was working. She was West Indian, mixed race, in her forties and good-looking with her hair in coiled plaits. She could just stand with the help of the nurses and could speak slurred words very slowly. It was her sense of humour that I remember most clearly. If anything funny happened – and it didn't take much for Joanne to find it funny – she would collapse in soundless laughter, her face creased, her mouth wide open. With this was a straightforward acknowledgment of her condition. I was touched by the way she accepted life. She didn't withdraw into a private darkness – even though she had good reason to do so – but stayed open and friendly. Somehow, she remained herself, with a quiet, unshowy courage and immense patience. One of the difficulties in working with patients with motor neurone disease is communication. Their speech can be very hard to understand and, if they try writing, this may be almost illegible because of the weakness in their arms and hands. This tests the patience not only of staff but also the patient herself in persevering in getting her message across when she can see those around do not understand her. I remember many occasions sitting with Joanne and us working out together what she wanted to say to me. This pared down our exchanges to the essentials. There could be no sophisticated dialogues on the meaning of suffering. My questions and comments needed to be short and clear so that she could respond in kind. Interestingly, these encounters had more depth to them than others I have had with patients who couldn't stop talking; their verbal flood was actually a barrier to communication.

Koan Time

Zen Buddhism has a fiendish tradition in which the Master sets his disciple a koan as part of his training. This is often in the form of a question, but it is a question that cannot be answered by the logical mind, only through an intuitive leap of enlightenment. Some strange and famous examples are: What is the sound of one hand clapping? Does a dog have the Buddha nature? What was your original face before you were born? The disciple goes away and meditates and returns from time to time to his Master with what he thinks is the answer. Almost certainly it is not and the poor disciple becomes more and more frustrated as his intellectual offerings are rejected. At last, at the end of his tether, he has a breakthrough and finds his true answer. To give a flavour of this bizarre process, there is the story of a Master who placed a newborn chick in a bottle and then fed it grain. Soon it was too large to get out through the neck of the bottle. The Master's question to his disciple was: How does the chick get out of the bottle? As usual, the hapless disciple battled with his question and became more and more frustrated at being told his answers were wrong. At last, one day he lost control of his feelings and, furious, he slapped his Master hard across his face. The Master smiled happily and said: "Now the chick has got out of the bottle."

The West has its koans as well. It's just that we don't recognise them as such. Some relate to illness or adversity: "Why me?" "Why do children have to suffer?" "What have I done to deserve this?" "Why is there so much evil in the world?" This is nitty-gritty stuff. No theological or philosophical abstractions here. This is about the reality of our human condition. Here is a story about loss and its acceptance I have adapted from the Buddhist tradition.

Seeds

There was once a young woman who lived in a village with her husband. She was beautiful and he was both rich and handsome. They loved each other deeply and they had a son, a three year old boy, who was their greatest joy. Every day the woman gave thanks for their good fortune.

One day, however, their son fell ill. It's just a fever, she told herself confidently. He'll be over it soon. But instead he became worse. She called the doctor, who prescribed herbs, but these didn't help. Uneasy now, she called the priest from the temple to say prayers over her child. In addition, she dressed their altar at home with fragrant yellow flowers and offerings of the most expensive food she could find in the market to the deity they worshipped. Surely he will get well now, she thought to herself. My prayers have always been answered before. But she felt anxious. That night, her son became yet more ill. He shook violently with a high fever. His teeth chattered and sweat poured from his small body. All night she stayed with him, wiping the sweat away and encouraging him to drink the sips of water which were all he could manage. She held his hand and, silently and desperately, prayed for his healing, while her husband watched, dumb with fear and sadness, in the shadows of the room.

Slowly, their dear son weakened. His skin became cold and pale, his grip on her hand weakened, his breathing slowed, and, just before dawn, he died. She looked at his still body uncomprehendingly. "This cannot be!" she said, and began to wail and tear her clothes. Then she collected herself: "No! He will live!" Her voice was raw from her keening. She wrapped her son in a sheet, snatched him up and ran to the physician. "You must have other medicines," she said to him breathlessly. "Please! Try anything." The doctor was not sympathetic. He felt for the child's pulse and then told her curtly: "He is dead. There is nothing more you can do."

As the sun rose, a perfect red disc in the soft, opalescent morning air, she ran to the temple, carrying her son with her. She did not hear the lowing of the cattle down by the river, or the sweet sound of the dawn chorus of birds. She didn't notice the pleasant coolness of the air, nor the dun dust clouds that her feet kicked up as she ran. She only knew one thing: her son must not die.

She ran to the temple priest and begged him to intercede with the gods to save her son. She would do anything, would accept any trial, would even offer her own life if only he could live. The priest looked at her: a wild-eyed woman, her hair dishevelled, her clothes torn, holding tightly to her burden. He knew he could not give her what she wanted, but he was a kindly man. He thought for a moment and then said: "There is a wandering holy man who is staying in a grove of pipal trees half a mile outside the village to the east. He calls himself an awakened one. He might be able to help you." Quickly she turned and, without even taking her leave, ran off to find the holy man. Her breath grew short and her chest hurt as she hurried out of the village. There was not a moment to lose. She dared not slacken now. There was hope.

She found the holy man sitting cross-legged and silent under one of the pipal trees. She approached him cautiously and respectfully. He was her only hope and she didn't want to antagonise him. He opened his eyes and smiled at her. She told him her story and begged him to bring life back to her son. He looked at her. She didn't see the compassion he felt for her, nor the tears that pricked his eyes. Fearful, she only saw his silence. "Please put your son on the ground," he said. She laid him down. The holy man leaned forward and gently placed his right hand on the little boy's brow while his left touched the ground. "I will help you," he said, looking again at the woman.

He cut short her stammered thanks and said that he needed some mustard seeds. "Oh, that's easy," she cried. "I have some at home. I'll fetch them immediately." "No," he said, "they must come from a household that has never experienced a loss, never experienced a death."

She looked at him, trembling, her eyes staring, her movements agitated. "All right. I will find them," she said. With that, she snatched up her son, his lifeless body now stiffening, and hurried back to the village. She came to the first dwelling, a poor hut. She explained she needed mustard seeds to help bring her son back to life. The woman of the house was sympathetic. "Of course," she said. "I'll fetch some." As she turned, the bereft mother asked shakily if anyone had died in this house. "Ah, yes," said the woman sadly, "my brother died here last year." Quickly, the mother took her child and went on to the next household. It was the same story. She visited house after house, some rich, some poor; it was always the same. There was not one family that had not experienced some loss. All through the heat of the day as the glaring sun beat down on her head she toiled, asking the same question at each dwelling. She tried to ignore the habitual dark vultures that wheeled high in the pale sky above the village.

By afternoon she was exhausted. Her movements were slowed and she felt she could hardly carry the dead weight of her son anymore. She came to the last house in the village. A young woman came to the door, about her own age. Yes, she had some mustard seeds. But: yes, her own daughter had died two years ago from snakebite. At this, the mother sank to the floor, overwhelmed. She could fight no longer. There was no one who had not had some loss in their life. She would never find the elusive mustard seeds.

The woman of the house knelt down beside her and held her as her body was wracked with sobs. "I know," her comforter said. "It is so hard. I was the same when my little daughter died." She held her for a long time.

The woman got up at last, thanked her consoler and walked wearily back to the holy man. This time she saw his compassion, saw his thinness, his threadbare clothes, his bowl and his staff. "Something like this has happened to you, hasn't it?" she said quietly. He bowed his head silently in response. Then he rose and said: "Come, we must go to the temple." The sun was low on the western horizon now as she walked silently beside him. They fetched her husband and, as the three made their way through the village, one by one the villagers came out of their dwellings and followed them.

Later, while she watched the flames of the funeral pyre consuming her son's body, she looked in wonder around her at the many people who had come out of respect for her and her husband's loss. She still felt the raw wound in her soul but she felt, too, her heart dilate in sympathy with the many stories of grief that she had heard that day. Then she looked for the holy man. She saw him in the distance. He was walking away, staff in hand, heading toward the next village.

The Beach

When I was young, my parents used to take us – that is myself and my brother and two sisters – to a beach in South Devon at the weekend. At first we used to drive down in a cramped old Ford Prefect, but we soon graduated to an exciting Rover 90, which meant it had 90 horsepower. As we drove I would drift into fantasies of 90 horses pulling our stately steed along. I would idly wonder, what exactly constituted the power of one horse? I imagined, for some reason, an Arab stallion. But then again it might have been a mustang or a shire horse.

It was a stony beach but, despite the drawback of the discomfort of walking on the stones in bare feet, it had its own charm. We would drive through the village and out along the road running parallel to the beach. There would be some old weather-beaten fishing boats drawn up just past where the houses ended. We would park and make our way to the beach. It descended in steep stony waves, an effect of the tidal patterns, I supposed. From where we sat I could see tall sandstone cliffs rising to east and west and could hear the gulls calling as they flew over their nesting sites on the cliff faces. To the east, a river ran down a wide, low, lush, green valley and flowed into the sea.

Somehow the sun was always shining when we went there and I remember sitting on the stones, warmed by the sun and looking at their variety. They had a slight hazy grittiness – the salt left behind when the seawater from the last high tide had evaporated. Some were the size of an ostrich egg, some no more than a centimetre in diameter. Their colours were varied – greys, white, black, terracotta, green – and often combined. I would find a white pebble with a black line bisecting it. Or there might be a stone, part russet and part grey, with a white line dividing the colours. There might be a grey stone stippled with black and white. And the shapes – oval, heart-shaped, circular, angular, cuboid or broken and serrated. If I put the stones in water and then took them out, they became brilliant, shining, jewel-like. I would lapse into a sort of dream as I played with them. Sometimes I would take a handful down to the water's edge and practise skipping them along the surface of the sea.

Scattered in between the stones would be a multiplicity of types of shells, some whole but many broken by their contact with the stones rolling in the waves. Occasionally I would even find a lozenge-shaped white cuttlebone, which we might take back for our budgerigar at home.

The water was usually very clear, and cold. The beach continued to step down steeply underwater so we either sat in the rush of the waves up the beach and listened to the sounds of stones under and out of the water rolling and tumbling and striking against each other or, if we ventured a few feet in, we would have to swim.

After swimming I would sit on the beach, warm up in the sun, look pensively out to sea and the seemingly infinite horizon and watch the occasional sailing boat or tanker passing by in the distance, small dots in the immensity of the sea. My thoughts would slow down and my consciousness let in the blue immensities of water and sky before me. For a little I became, like them, still and timeless.

And then, one day, many years later when I was a teenager, I came across this passage written by Sir Isaac Newton shortly before he died:

I do not know what I may appear to the world, but to myself I seem to have been only like a boy playing on the seashore, and diverting myself in now and then finding a smoother pebble or a prettier shell than ordinary, whilst the great ocean of truth lay all undiscovered before me.
(Brewster 1855 p. 407)

I knew that place; I had been there, as for that matter had countless thousands of others. I had sat playing with pebbles and shells and, musing, looked out too at that great undiscovered ocean. Now I had also wrestled at school with Newton's laws of motion and universal gravitation and the abstractions of calculus. Those words above, however, brought me closer in a few moments to the man than all my school studies. What a humble thing for such a great scientist to say.

I remember once having an echocardiogram, an investigation in which ultrasound waves are bounced off the various surfaces of the heart to produce a picture of it in action. When the technician had finished the scan, she showed me a recording of it in real time which, moreover, was in colour. I watched my heart beating with fascination and growing wonder. I could see every chamber. I could watch them contracting and relaxing ceaselessly and see the heart valves rhythmically opening and closing. What impressed me was how mobile, how bouncy, these chambers were. It seemed as though they were dancing to a Latin American rhythm – a salsa perhaps. And all of this went on without my even thinking about it. It's true there have been remarkable advances in diagnosis and treatment of heart conditions but, for me, they do not compare with the awe I felt watching my own heart beating. Before my very eyes, life was unfolding. I was gazing at Newton's great undiscovered ocean.

Chapter 10

Love

Doctors don't talk about love, at least not that I've ever heard. They might be all right with words like care or compassion, conscientiousness or competence, duty or ethics, but love, no. It would be like belching in church: not done.

Dr Albert Schweitzer, however, got close. He was sitting musing on the deck of a barge chugging along an African river and through a herd of submerged hippopotamuses, when the phrase "Reverence for Life" popped unexpectedly into his head. This aphorism encapsulated his approach as a medical missionary working in the hospital, Lambarené, that he had built in Gabon, West Africa, following his arrival there in 1913. Something of the meaning of this motto can be discerned from his description of operating on a patient with a strangulated hernia, which was a much-dreaded illness among Africans at the time. Since surgery was not available before he came, the dire course of events was as follows: the intestines, being obstructed, swelled and the abdomen became grossly and painfully distended from gas. After some days, the guts would rupture and the spilling of their contents into the cavity of the abdomen caused excruciating pain and a slow agonising death.

Schweitzer commented: "But that I can save him from days of torture, that is what I feel as my great and ever new privilege. Pain is a more terrible lord of mankind than even death itself." Here is his description of what happened after he had operated on a local African for this illness:

The operation is finished, and in the hardly-lighted dormitory, I watch for the sick man's awaking. Scarcely has he recovered consciousness when he stares about him and ejaculates again

and again: "I've no more pain! I've no more pain!" His hand feels for mine and will not let it go... The African sun is shining through the coffee bushes into the dark shed, but we, black and white, sit side by side and feel that we know by experience the meaning of the words: "And all ye are brethren"(Matt. xxiii, 8).
(Schweitzer 1948, pp. 62–3)

Any doctor would resonate with what Schweitzer described, that extraordinary feeling that comes from saving the life of a fellow human being.

There is, though, another transcendent dimension to love in its healing capacity. Here is a description by a doctor, a friend, who wrote this account for me of an experience she had. She has agreed to it being included here but prefers to remain anonymous:

I had come into work early so that I would have time to meditate before I did my ward rounds. I was feeling despondent that morning and not relishing the prospect of seeing a ward full of dying people. I had the familiar frustrating feeling of struggling to maintain concentration while I meditated, a distracted, scattered feeling. I remember focusing once more on my breathing and then, suddenly and unexpectedly, becoming aware of light all around me, although my eyes were closed. I felt my whole being taken up by this light. It seemed rich, white, with the slightest hint of gold and was very beautiful. My inner experience was transformed. I felt alive, filled with the experience of love. It was so intense I wondered if I would be able to bear it, but I didn't want it to stop. I don't know how long it went on, perhaps a few minutes. When it receded, my despondency had gone and I felt an awakeness and appreciation of the beauty of ordinary things around me. My ward round was transformed.

I seemed to be able to see the patients much more clearly and sense their emotional temperature. Talking with them I didn't feel the familiar sense of not being able to do enough to meet their needs. I felt no heaviness in being with the dying. It seemed a few minutes was enough to engage deeply and communicate what needed to be communicated. As we talked, compassion and love were my main experiences. During the next couple of days or so, a sort of afterglow of the light would come back from time to time. On reflection, it seems to me that what I experienced felt more real, more true, more alive than our circumscribed, dull ordinary reality.

Meeting

"A person is a person because of people." So goes a traditional Zulu saying which highlights a fundamental aspect of our existence, namely that it is *always* relational, whether this be with other people, with the different aspects of ourselves, with nature or with a deity. So much of the distress I have seen in the dying is about some unresolved conflict in one of their relationships. It might, too, have been about the loneliness of those who live a solitary widowed life; or it might have been an unfulfilled longing to have had children.

The destructive effects of lack of relationship are particularly obvious in children who have been neglected. I remember being struck by a film called *The Wild Child*, directed by François Truffaut, which I saw in 1970 when I was still a medical student. It is based on the true story of Victor of Aveyron, a feral child in 18th century France who had apparently lived his whole life in the woods. When found he was naked and had multiple scars on his body, including one across his throat. He ate acorns and roots. He behaved like a wild animal, biting and scratching anyone that crossed him, and showing no signs of interaction with other children. He hated confinement. He was insensitive to cold and would pick potatoes out of boiling water and eat them with no sign of pain. He was thought to be about twelve years old. A medical student, Jean Itard, took him in and tried to civilise him. He did make some progress over the years, but Victor's understanding of language was only ever rudimentary and he never comprehended tones of voice. He did, however, show some affection for his carers. Itard (1802, p. 75) wrote:

If I go to his chamber, in the evening, when he is about to retire to rest, the first thing that he does is to prepare himself for my embrace; then he draws me to him, by laying hold of my arm, and making me sit on his bed. Then in general he seizes my hand, draws it over his eyes, his forehead, and the back part of his head, and detains it with his own, a long time, applied to those parts.

Despite Itard's strenuous efforts, Victor was never able to develop anything like the full range of social interactions normal for any child. There is, however, a beautiful scene in the film when Victor joyfully scampers out at night on to the lawn in front of Itard's house, sometimes on all fours. Then he looks up, becomes still and stares at the moon, entranced. Somehow, despite his sufferings, his humanity, his personhood, has not been destroyed.

Martin Buber was a philosopher who brought about a revival in Hasidic Jewish mysticism. He thought deeply about relationships and described two attitudes. One is of *I* in relation to *It* which is like the connection between subject and object – me and my car, you and your watch and so on. The other is of *I* and *Thou*. Here, relationship is of such a profundity that the separateness of *I* and *It* gives way to the oneness of a meeting of depths, a meeting of souls. Buber had a recurring dream, which he called the dream of the double cry, that symbolised this theme powerfully (Buber 1961, pp. 17–19).

He would be in a primitive world, in a vast cave, a mud building or a gigantic forest. Something extraordinary would happen to him; for example a small animal resembling a lion cub would tear at the flesh of his arm and would have to be forced to desist. This part of the dream would unfold rapidly, but then the pace would slow. "I stand there and cry out," he writes. This cry would be "sometimes joyous, sometimes fearful, sometimes even filled with both pain and with triumph." It is "inarticulate but in strict rhythm, rising and falling, swelling to a fullness which my throat could not endure were I awake, long and slow, quiet, quite slow and very long, a cry that is a song." Then, "far away, another cry moves towards me, another which is the same… sung by another voice. Yet it is not the same cry… but rather its true rejoinder." It seemed to Buber his cry was a series of questions to which the reply was a response. And then a "true dream certitude comes to me that *now it has happened*."

What was the dream referring to? Simply this: it is in our authentic encounter with one another, which we call love, that we become alive. I become I through my encounter with You. It is relevant, too, that it is an experience of suffering that leads to Buber's initial cry and this in turn evokes a response from the Other.

In these *I-Thou* encounters, it is as though a field is created between the participants encompassing them both. Such a relationship may occur not just with people, but with any other thing, whether animate or inanimate. I recall many hospice inpatients who pined for their pets and were as full of joy when they were brought in for a visit as if they had been a long-lost relative. Victor, the wild child, was entranced by the moon.

When we were staying in Port Douglas, we met an Australian surgeon called Harry, who had decided to take a year out from his surgical training and go walkabout. He told us of how when he was out walking in the bush, he came across a forested mountain. There was a path leading upwards with the usual signs for tourists giving a history and geography of the place. Just by the path was a sign put up by the Aboriginal tribe that lived in that area. It said that this was a sacred mountain, a manifestation of a Dreaming spirit. The sign requested visitors not to climb the mountain. Just then a group of sturdy white Australians, shod in walking boots and carrying backpacks, strode purposefully off up the path ignoring the printed request. For them, the mountain and forest were an *It*, an object to be conquered. But for the Aborigines, the mountain was alive, a *Thou*. To walk on it was to tread on sacred ground. This is a familiar biblical theme. When Moses saw the burning bush on

Mount Horeb, God instructed him to take off his shoes because he was on holy ground.

Harry was in a dilemma. He wanted to climb the mountain but the ancestral owners asked visitors not to. He felt strongly about respecting aboriginal rights so he decided on an experiment: he would treat the mountain as if it were a Dreaming spirit, just as they did. He silently asked permission to enter the forest trail. He said he had no idea who or what he might be talking to or what the reply might be. In response he had, to his surprise, a clear sense of permission – but he was not to take any photographs. The whole tone of his walk altered after this. It was, he said, rather like being in cathedral. Quietness and respect were needed. Instead of religious paintings and statues, he had the buttressed trees soaring up to the sky. Instead of altars there were ancient stones covered with moss. As I listened to his story, I thought the wild boy, Victor, would have been at home there.

Le Général

Often, we only discover fragments of stories. I recall, as a junior doctor, looking after a French Foreign Legion general, who had advanced cancer. A dignified man, he looked the part, with silver hair cut short *en brosse*, white stubble on a determined chin and a resolute expression. But it was clear from what he told me in his strong French accent that he had been struggling to cope because of pain and increasing weakness. His English partner reminded me of a 1920s flapper. Although elderly, she presented herself as young. She wore her white hair in a bob and had applied thick mascara and bright red lipstick. Her flamboyant hat and dress seemed to come from an earlier time. She was an extrovert and talked unceasingly in her upper class accent about how she could no longer look after her partner, whom she obviously adored, at home because of his deteriorating condition. I was touched by their closeness. However, behind her bright façade, she was clearly very distressed. She could have stepped out of an Evelyn Waugh novel, or she might have been a character in a story about the British Raj in India. She pressed me to take some money. I sensed resonances of years of tipping people to get the best service. I felt compassionate more than embarrassed. I refused as gently as I could. It was the only way she had left to her in her desperate quest to help her partner. He died within a few days and I never did have an opportunity find out more of their past life and how they met, though I was very curious about them – I wanted to know how they fitted together, I wanted to make sense of their unusual partnership. I felt as if I had walked into a theatre during the final few minutes of a play, the death scene, and had no idea how the characters had arrived there.

Ruby

Ruby was in her eighties when I met her. She had been a dancer and used to perform at the notorious Windmill Theatre during the Second World War. I don't know if she took part in their famous nude tableaux – the participants were required to be still to get past the censor – but I wouldn't put it past her. She settled in to her four-bedded bay in the hospice and held court to her many visitors. She wore silk, flared, champagne-coloured pyjamas and a silk turban to hide her thinning hair. She had retained her 1940s BBC cut-glass accent, though it was sometimes slurred by her intake of gin – three-quarters of a bottle a day along with a sniff or two of tonic water. Champagne was produced regularly by her friends and this was added to her usual intake of spirits. There was something of the feel of a time warp when she partied with her cronies. We might have been backstage at the Windmill Theatre after a performance, watching the cast letting their hair down in a haze of cigarette smoke accompanied by the clinking of glasses and loud laughter. I liked her style.

She presented a prescribing problem for me since I had to be cautious of the dose of morphine I gave her for her pain in case it interacted with her alcohol and led to excessive sedation. By careful titration of her analgesia we were able to arrive at a satisfactory level of pain control without her falling asleep all the time.

Ruby refused all attempts to explore how she felt about having advanced cancer and the prospect of dying, and it became evident that gin was her answer to such issues. This was most apparent if another patient in the bay became more ill or died. Ruby's daily gin intake would increase in line with the seriousness of that patient's condition, peaking at one and a quarter bottles. She simply became rather drowsier, more slurred, and swayed more obviously when she was sitting up. Next day she would be fine.

Weren't we colluding with her heavy drinking? Yes, we were. Shouldn't we have been detoxing her? Absolutely not. It would have meant putting her through a stressful procedure only to have her die maybe a week or two later. That would have been cruel. She was never an aggressive drunk. This was the way she had chosen and she wasn't going to change.

I wonder what had happened in her life to cause her to blot it out with gin. A broken marriage? A lover killed during the war? Perhaps, too, she remembered dancing in the Windmill Theatre while German bombs fell all around them, and experiencing the powerful rush of aliveness in extreme danger, in facing death and surviving. These were past times, the most intense in her life, times to which she could never return. Maybe it was easier to stay in a time warp than mourn what was gone.

I like to think she is in a place where she no longer needs a bottle of gin to ease her sorrows, where her hurts are healed and where there is lots of dancing.

The Bikers

When Mary was admitted to the hospice where I was working in Hertfordshire, we soon discovered that she was a member of a bikers' chapter. Her visitors were big, powerful men, some with shoulder-length hair, long moustaches and grizzled beards. They wore studded black leather jackets with the name and logo of their group on the back and carried their crash helmets with, if memory serves, an eagle logo on them. Their partners came too, in similar gear. Huge motorbikes, some Harley-Davidsons, gleaming black and silver, were parked outside.

I was, at first, anxious. How would we manage these visitors, I wondered. Images of aggressive Hell's Angels came to mind. It turned out, though, that I was completely wrong. They were actually like a big extended family and looked out for each other. There were always two or three of them sitting with Mary and her biker partner in her room. They would take turns, knowing that too many visitors would be more than Mary could take on, and not wanting to disturb the routine of the ward either. They were thoughtful, courteous and kind, the complete antithesis of my preconceptions about bikers.

They wanted to support the hospice too. Some time later, after Mary had died, they attended the lighting of a Christmas tree outside as part of a fund-raising drive. It was night and staff and patients were looking out from the brightly lit ward into the darkness, while crowds of visitors stood on the lawn in front of the tree. Just as the tree lights were lit I heard a throaty roar and, looking to my left, I saw a row of half a dozen motorbikes with their biker riders, who were gunning the engines and shining their headlights on to the tree.

I shall never look at a biker in the same way again.

The Wedding

From time to time there have been marriages in the different hospices I've worked in. Mostly, these have been very quiet affairs: the Registrar, the couple and one or two family members at most. Some have taken place a matter of days before a patient's death.

Juliet, however, was an exception. The first thing that struck me about her was her beauty. When she came to see me in outpatients I could not have told by looking at her that she had recurrent cancer causing considerable pain. She had long, blond hair with highlights, and grey-blue eyes. She was tall and fashionably dressed and the vivacity of her personality came over immediately. Her partner, Andrew, quieter than her, accompanied her. He was a barrister. From the beginning, her pain was unusually difficult to keep under control. I would try one combination of drugs which worked for a while and then the pain would reassert itself. It was a neuropathic pain, that is one where the cancer invades the nerves themselves, rendering them exquisitely hypersensitive. During all this time, she retained her sense of humour and her ability to relate even when she was in pain.

One day, she was admitted for pain control to the London hospice where I was working. It was during this time that she and Andrew decided to get married – and they wanted a proper wedding. What I remember most was how the hospice staff helped them to achieve this. She had bought an intricate lace wedding dress and veil. The nurses helped her with all her preparations – hair, nails, make-up, her bouquet, a photographer. She wanted her pain medicines to be kept at as low a dose as possible so that she would be alert. That day she seemed to outface her pain. Somehow, she looked well, even though I knew the extent of her illness and its effects on her. With Andrew and their three children, she was able to manage the short car journey to the church nearby. Their photographs show a beautiful bride with her husband, in a sense just like a thousand other photographs of beautiful brides, except that in Juliet's case, she had, for that day, risen above the illness that was her hidden companion.

Chapter 11

Transformation

As a junior doctor I used to work for a plastic surgeon. He was a plain-speaking no-nonsense man, an expert in operations on cancers of the head and neck which often required plastic surgery as well. More often, however, he did cosmetic surgery, enlarging or reducing breasts, and doing facelifts, tummy tucks and the like. I suppose those operated on hoped their lives would be transformed as if a change on the surface could somehow change them within. I was rather doubtful.

In real transformations, change happens from the inside, just as caterpillars inside their cocoon metamorphose into butterflies. This change is a recurring theme in myths and fairy tales. Wooden Pinocchio is changed into a real boy. The Beast in *Beauty and the Beast* is transformed into a handsome prince when Belle falls in love with him and kisses him. The Ugly Duckling turns out to be a beautiful swan.

These stories reflect our own life transformations of birth, childhood, adolescence, adulthood, retirement, bereavement and death. Each of these liminal events changes us in some way.

Imagine being born and the loss of your warm and comfortable womb with its reassuring steady heartbeat, the terrible pressure of the contracting uterus, the sudden onslaught of dazzling lights and loud noises, your terror, your feeling of asphyxiation only relieved by your first breath, the cold air on your skin, the giant hands that pick you up, the soothing contact, skin to skin, with your mother and her comforting breast. This is an epic, transforming journey indeed.

Imagine living with the possibility of a violent death every day, living on the edges of life. This is what happened to Corrie ten Boom, a Dutch woman who was imprisoned in Ravensbrück concentration camp during the Second World War, a place of starvation, illness, brutality and mass murder. Through an administrative error she was released near the end of the war. She suffered from malnutrition, her limbs were swollen, she was dressed in rags, and was filthy and ridden with lice. It was winter and she made her way in the bitter cold slowly towards Holland. She was taken in by a Christian hospital and for the first time in years was greeted with kindness. Her appearance was so changed that the nurse, who was an acquaintance of hers, did not recognise her at first. Food appeared. Corrie writes: "'I have never seen anyone eat so intensely,' one of the nurses from a nearby table commented. I cared not. With every mouthful of food I could feel new life streaming into my body... Then came a warm bath. They could hardly get me out of it." Next she was dressed for bed. "I felt so happy that I laughed for sheer joy. How sweet they were to me." She was taken to her bedroom. "How lovely was the combination of colours. I was starved for colour. In the concentration camp, everything was grey... And the bed! Delightfully soft and clean with thick woollen blankets... I wanted to laugh and cry at the same time." There were books, and she could hear the whistle of a canal boat, the sounds of little children, of a choir and of a carillon. "I closed my eyes and tears wet my pillow. Only to those who have been in prison does freedom have such a great meaning." (ten Boom 2005, pp. 23–6)

This is a kind of rebirth or even resurrection experience, and it was accompanied by a transformation in her life after the war. Formerly a watchmaker she toured the world speaking of her experiences in concentration camp and how her faith had brought her through. It was a message of hope and of freedom.

Dying, of course, is a time of transformation as well:

The clear morning sun shines through the windows. I part the curtains around the bed and step into another world. The light from outside is softened and diffused by the screen. An old woman with white hair lies in the bed, her eyes closed. She has died peacefully during the night. An atmosphere of indescribable tranquillity fills the space about her. I have been called by the hospice nurses, who hold her in special affection, to certify that she has died. I feel calmness diffuse into me like a tide as I listen to her still heart. I think to myself that, wherever she is, she is in a good place. The experience stays with me for the rest of that day.

There is a beautiful Sufi story on this theme about a wonderful bird called the Simurgh. He is the king of the birds. No one has ever seen him. The only evidence of his existence is a famed and wonderful feather dropped from his wing far away in China. All the birds speak together in a parliament and, longing to know who the Simurgh is, decide they will seek him out guided by the hoopoe. The journey is long and hard and, one by one, they drop out. They must cross seven perilous valleys and by the time they reach the Simurgh's holy mountain only thirty birds are left. Purified by their suffering they discover a lake and gaze at its mirror-like surface. They see themselves and suddenly realise that the Simurgh indwells each of them and all of them. He is their transcendent truth, the God within. (Attar 1984)

The Woman in the Ambulance

The Accident and Emergency Department in St George's Hospital, Tooting in South London was, at the time I worked there around thirty years ago, a conglomeration of pre-fabricated single-storey buildings. It had that air of scruffiness that you often find in older NHS buildings – scuffed paint, misshapen rubber swing doors with scratched plastic windows, notices posted everywhere, worn linoleum, the smell of hospital disinfectant. In short, it had character. One day, we received a call from an ambulance crew. They were bringing in a "cardiac arrest", a woman who had been in a car accident and had received severe head injuries. We readied ourselves. Normally, the crew would rush in pushing their charge on a stretcher – speed was essential. This time, they called me out to the ambulance; they felt, as they put it, that this woman was a "goner". Ambulance crews normally try very hard to resuscitate just about every patient they are called to who has collapsed, so I knew they would have good reason for their pessimism.

I climbed into the ambulance and felt it rocking as I walked along the narrow gap between the stretcher slots on the left, and to the right where my patient lay. She was a young good-looking woman with long, dark hair and still dressed in the dark browns and greens she had chosen that morning. I looked at her. Her mouth was slightly open and her sightless eyes stared up at the ceiling of the ambulance. Dark blood seeped from the back of her head, but otherwise there were no apparent signs of injury. I felt an immediate certainty that she was irrevocably dead and that her skull was cracked like an egg. This might seem too obvious even to state, but it was not a scientific opinion based on examination. It was more of an intuitive perception – a different dimension of knowing. I examined her: no breath sounds, no heartbeat, fixed dilated pupils. I looked into the fundi of her eyes.

I could see the arteries and veins of the retina branching like trees. Only now the arteries no longer looked like smooth tubes, but instead were constricted in segments. This is known as rail-roading since it looks like sequences of tracks on a rail line and is a sign of cessation of blood flow due to cardiac arrest. My rational conclusion was clearly the same: death, certified at such and such a time. And yet... as I recall I also had a clear impression that she was still present in some way and, further, that she was in shock. Of course, it made no sense to hold two apparently contradictory perceptions and I made nothing further of it at the time.

Some years later, my eye was caught by an advert. Sogyal Rinpoche a Tibetan lama would be giving a talk at Regent's Park College to coincide with the publication of his book, *The Tibetan Book of Living and Dying*. I decided to go; the hall was packed. There was an introductory speaker, a warm-up man. To my surprise, John Cleese strode on to the stage. I recall feeling rather disappointed since he insisted on being serious, but it said something about the respect he had for Sogyal Rinpoche that he was prepared to help in this way. Then the lama himself appeared. He was a short, round, jolly man with a frequent high-pitched laugh. He spoke fast and in explosive bursts. As I took in his presence, I had the curious impression of a powerful energy flowing through him. I found his talk inspiring. He spoke of his culture – one that accepted death as part of life, and believed in each person preparing for their end. He commented on how shocked he was to find such a culture of denial around death in the West. At the end of the talk, I bought his book.

When I read it, I came across descriptions of what Tibetans call the bardo states. These include the experiences of a person after death. One passage caught my eye. It spoke of those who have undergone a violent, sudden or distressing death. The author suggested that the dying person may become imprisoned in the painful experience of his death and unable to let go.

(Rinpoche 1992) His body is dead but he is trapped. He may not even realise he is dead.

A few years ago, an unusual situation arose in a hospice where I was working. Several staff had heard voices and moans in the lift shaft at times when they knew the lift was empty. One of the junior doctors also told me that he had experienced objects such as pencils moving spontaneously on his desk. The chaplain was very clear about what was happening. This was, she said, the soul of a person who had died in the hospice who did not realise that she was dead. She was trapped in the moment of death. Was this, I wondered, an example of the bardo state that I had read about years before? The chaplain proposed a service to help release this soul and invited me to attend. I had never encountered this before and I was curious about what would happen.

My main memory of the service is one of light – there were candles and a bowl of water in which floated yellow flowers. It also had a lightness to it – it wasn't the weighty affair that I expected. During the service, the chaplain prayed for the dead person, telling her very simply that she had died and it was time to release her hold on this life and to continue on her journey.

There were no more voices or moving objects after the service.

Perhaps this was what I had noticed when I attended the young woman in the ambulance. Perhaps she had been trapped similarly by the violence and suddenness of her death. If I am right, I hope that, whatever the funeral rituals were that her family had arranged, these, too, would have had the effect of setting her free.

Fire! Fire!

I was talking with a group of hospice staff once when one of them told this story. It was about a terminally ill man who was a devout Buddhist. During his final illness, he continued his meditation practice. One day he became very agitated. He called out repeatedly that he was on fire. The hospice nurses tried to calm him, thinking that he was confused and hallucinating. He continued to cry out, seemingly in distress. They tried everything they knew to help him. They even had the ingenious idea of pouring water over him to persuade him that the fire had been put out, but unfortunately to no avail. He died not long afterwards.

Later, they learned of the Fire Buddha – Indian depictions of the Buddha sometimes show him as a pillar of fire. We cannot now say with certainty what this man was experiencing, but the hypothesis that, as he meditated in preparation for his death, he identified with the Fire Buddha to the extent of experiencing this in his sensory body, is a possibility. While knowledge of Buddhist meditative states would have been helpful, perhaps the most important lesson here is of seeing with beginner's eyes, of being open to explanations or diagnoses outside the usual run of things. In this account, there was perhaps a confusion of levels – what was thought to be a psychophysical pathology may have been a mystical state not amenable to fire extinguishers.

At the Frontier

The closest I have ever got to a near-death experience was when I was ironing. It was an old iron with parts of the plastic cladding cracked or missing. I had touched the iron's surface to feel if it was hot enough. This was a mistake. My left hand, holding the handle, was, unknown to me, touching a live wire sticking out through the cladding. When my right hand touched the iron, a circuit was completed, my arm and hand muscles went into spasm and I could feel the current juddering through me at 50 cycles per second. Somehow I eventually dropped the iron and fell to the ground, feeling as though I had been hit by lightning, which in a sense I had. My whole body tingled as if a fire had swept through it. My heart pounded so hard that I wondered if it might stop, overwhelmed by the energy bolts it had received.

Perhaps I should have felt grateful to be alive after this close encounter of an electrical kind. Actually I felt frightened and angry. I had recently become engaged and my life was going well. How could such a potentially fatal accident occur now? It seemed so unfair. I felt the fragility of life and how little control any of us have over our lives. Later on, ill and dying people were often to voice similar feelings to me. It took me a week to recover some equilibrium – I was lucky though; I got better.

Others, however, have gone further – they have crossed over and returned to tell the tale. Since a doctor, RA Moody, first described in 1976 examples of patients who had died, been resuscitated and then, on returning to consciousness, told of visiting the afterlife during their near-death experience, there have been a library of writings on this subject. There is one example that I have found particularly moving. The origins of this go back to when I was working as a doctor in a mining village in Northern Manitoba in Canada. It, and the open cast mine it served, were set in a vast wilderness of conifers, rivers and lakes. The nearest town was 135 miles away. The health centre provided care for the miners and their families and also for the local Native Canadian Indians – there was a reservation not far away.

I soon became aware of the plight of the Indians – dispossessed from their traditional lands, distanced from their culture, numbing their pain with alcohol – their experience was, like that of their American cousins, one of soul loss. One incident highlighted this for me. A Native Canadian was brought into the Emergency Room. He was in his forties, with long, black hair tied back in a ponytail and his face was burnt by his outdoors life. He swayed and staggered as he walked. His speech was slurred and he smelt strongly of alcohol. There was a bloodstain seeping through the clothes of his left upper arm. He had been out trapping and had caught a beaver. He was using the butt of his rifle to kill it. He was so drunk that he accidently pulled the trigger as he brought the rifle down on the beaver's head. The bullet lodged in the man's shoulder near a major artery. We had to send him by air to the nearest town with surgical facilities. It seemed ironic that he was engaged in hunting, an important part of the traditions of his people, and at the same time drinking, an import from European colonists. It was as though he was shooting himself in the foot – only for him it was the shoulder.

Some years later, I came across a book called *Black Elk Speaks*, which caught my attention because of my experiences in Canada. The author, John Neihardt (1988), was interested in the Native American Indian way of life and, in 1930, had acted as a scribe taking down the spoken words of Black Elk, a holy man of the Oglala Sioux, as translated by his son. It was a moving story, imbued with sadness – Black Elk lived through the Battle of Little Bighorn in 1876 and the Wounded Knee Massacre in 1890. He saw his people driven from their traditional lands, corralled in reservations and forced to go to mission schools. Nevertheless the words of Black Elk have been an inspiration to his nation. Perhaps most famous is a vision, part of a near-death experience he had when he was nine years old. He had been "... sick for twelve days, lying like dead all the while." As he lay in his tepee, he saw two men with flaming spears coming from the clouds. They stood nearby and called: "'Hurry! Come! Your Grandfathers are calling you!'" A cloud came down and bore him up to the sky. There followed an extraordinary and complex vision prophetic of the sufferings of the Sioux people and indeed of the whole world, but with an ultimate message of hope. Remarkably, the Tree of Life makes an appearance:

> ... I looked ahead and saw the mountains there with rocks and forest on them, and from the mountains flashed all colours upward to the heavens. Then I was standing on the highest mountain of them all, and round about beneath me was the whole hoop of the world. And while I stood there I saw more than I can tell and I understood more than I saw; for I was seeing in a sacred manner the shapes of all things in the spirit, and the shape of all shapes as they must live together like one being. And I saw that the sacred hoop of my people was one of many hoops that made one circle, wide as daylight and as starlight, and in the centre grew one mighty flowering tree to shelter all the children of one mother and one father. And I saw it was holy.
> (Neihardt 1988, p. 43)

The Inner Tyre

As far as I know, no one else has commandeered an inner tyre for quite this use. My sister was very young at the time, perhaps three or four years old. We had recently moved to a house in Devon, a large white one with lots of rooms, stairs, a cellar and an attic to explore. But, even better, it had a big garden shaded by two large copper beeches which made for excellent climbing practice. There was a walnut tree in which my brother later built a tree platform and a coop with hens at the bottom of the garden, a relic of the Second World War and rationing when their great-grandhen mothers provided a welcome supply of free eggs. The hens mysteriously disappeared sometime after we moved in; I never quite worked out where they went, though I suspect into the oven.

I don't know where my sister found the black rubber inner tyre but she used to take it out on to the lawn, put it down, and then sit cross-legged in it gazing into the distance. It seemed to me she did this for hours, though it was probably much less since I had a child's view of time which hung heavy on me whenever anything was boring. She most certainly didn't want to be disturbed when I tapped her on the shoulder. At the time I was rather annoyed by her unavailability to play games. This solitary 'game' of hers was such a feature that a neighbour even did a watercolour of her sitting there surrounded by apple trees in her self-created circle – a Garden of the Hesperides, perhaps.

In hindsight it seems clear to me. Children have a natural propensity to enter a meditative state, something which is often drilled out of them. ("Stop daydreaming!" say their parents, teachers, tutors, sergeant majors and managers.) This unpremed-itated meditation was, I think, what my sister was doing. She sat cross-legged, a common meditative posture, and she placed herself within a ring, a symbol of wholeness, of body and soul in communion. She wasn't taught to do this; it wasn't part of any religious training. She just wanted to. As far as I can tell, my parents had no idea of what she was doing. I wonder if they might have stopped her if they had realised. As it was, she was left to her spontaneous spiritual practice.

There is another aspect to this story. There is an ancient symbol in Greek and Egyptian mythology, the Ouroboros or world snake, which is portrayed as a serpent coiled in a circle having swallowed its tail. It represents, among other things, the conservation of energy in an individual, the protection of life within which may be threatened by big changes such as the move to a new house which my sister experienced. She instinctively formed a protective circle around her. As I look back and remember this story, I find myself wanting to go back to the past and say to that little girl: "Good for you."

Children, then, have a spiritual life whether they are brought up within a religious tradition or not. I came across an example of this, in the context of illness, a touching story about a courageous child called Nick, who died of cancer when he was nine. (Byrne 2008, p. 254)

> ... he got his parents to bring him back to see me. He insisted on seeing me alone and told his parents that they must stay in the car, that he needed to see me without them. When we were on our own, Nick told me that he talked to his guardian angel all the time... his angel had told him that in the future, maybe soon, he would be taking him to Heaven. Nick said that was OK with him, that he was nine years of age now... he had told his Mum and Dad that he would be going to Heaven someday soon, but they had replied that they didn't want to hear that kind of talk.

Some might say that Nick was hallucinating and deluded. To me, he actually sounded rather sane. He was prepared to face the fact that he would soon die, he knew that his parents couldn't cope with this and he didn't want to hurt their feelings. I thought he showed considerable insight and resilience, not to mention courage. We are then left with the unsettling but exhilarating possibility that he was simply telling the truth.

Orana

There is a painting by Paul Gauguin which is not quite what it seems. At first nothing appears unusual. The setting, as usual for Gauguin, is Tahiti. We can see coconut trees and other flowering tropical trees. There is a volcanic mountain in the background and a clearing with open-sided huts. In the foreground, near a table carrying bowls of tropical fruits, is a beautiful young Tahitian woman. Barefoot, she wears a sarong calf-length and tucked in place just above her breast. The dress is red with large white flowers on it. Her naked son, who is perhaps three or four years old, is sitting on her left shoulder so that his left leg dangles down between her breasts and his right down her back. His body leans against the left side of her head, and his head has fallen forward on to the crown of her head. He has turned his own head to look shyly out at the viewer. It is an image of intimacy. Two adolescent girls, bare-breasted as was the custom then in Tahiti, are looking on, and behind them walks another Tahitian woman, half-hidden by a flowering plant, her face turned away from the viewer's gaze.

It is at this point that we encounter something strange – the woman has wings, blue, yellow-gold and purple wings. She is, in fact, an angel – and a Tahitian angel at that. She is holding a long curving golden feather. Her bare feet seem to be lifted slightly off the ground. Then we see that the hands of the two adolescent girls are steepled, palms together, in prayer. Furthermore, the mother and child each have a fine circle of gold around their heads. They are sancti, holy.

This, then, is a picture of Mary and her child, Jesus. By portraying them as Tahitian in a Tahitian setting, Gauguin has thrown us out of our usual frame of reference. The familiar Mary of European paintings, looking distinctly Flemish, dressed in gorgeous embroidered robes of gold and scarlet and blue, attended by the Three Kings bringing lavish gifts of gold, frank-incense and myrrh, while energetic golden-haired angels play viols and sackbuts, has gone. Nor is there a chubby, pink, baby Jesus with flaxen curls and blue eyes, already able to sit up despite being newborn. Instead we have real people painted from life, in a tropical setting utterly different from our Northern European historical portrayals of the childhood of Jesus. He and his mother are flesh-and-blood, sensual, connected skin to skin. Suddenly the human, physical reality of an ordinary young woman called Miryam and her son called Yeshua comes home to us. We can see their closeness with fresh eyes, we can understand that they loved each other just as any mother and child would nowadays.

This painting restores the body with its sensual aliveness to its proper place in the world of the sacred. Gauguin called it *La Orana Maria*, or *Hail Mary*.

Chapter 12

Another Country

There is a way that we live in two countries at once. One, of course, is the physical geography we inhabit. The other, we only catch a glimpse of from time to time. We see it in the eyes of a child studying a leaf with intense, innocent attention, or of a baby staring rapt at the play of light on a ceiling. We see it in that faraway look people have when they dive into an inner world of mythic images, or when they meditate or pray. We hear its sounds in music. We read of it in poetry. The scent of a flower will suddenly transport us to this other place. Or it may appear suddenly and unbidden when we least expect it: seeing "a world in a grain of sand," as William Blake (1994 p. 135) put it. We fall in love and our loved one is, for a while, transformed into something like a divine figure. And we may encounter it when we are dying.

Being Reconciled

He was quite young, in his fifties, pale, dark-haired and ill. He had advanced cancer and was convinced that the Devil was waiting to carry him off to Hell. I remember his restlessness, his wide eyes and pupils so dilated that his eyes looked black, along with a pressured quality to the way he spoke. His agitation and fear were obvious. I myself felt an uneasiness talking to him. Perhaps I was osmotically picking up his distress. I wondered if this might be the early stages of a paranoid psychosis, and I was concerned lest he enter into an acutely disturbed state. He was, however, able to talk with and listen to members of staff on his hospice ward and he obviously found comfort in doing so, but his fears and a sense of dread would soon return when he was left alone. He was a Roman Catholic and asked to see a priest, which we arranged. He decided to make a confession – there were issues in his life about which he felt much guilt. After he had done so, his distress subsided and did not return. He died peacefully a couple of days later.

What was happening here? Was this a psychiatric condition – a delusional psychosis? If so, it seems very unlikely that his confession which, after all, is not a standard psychiatric intervention would have allayed his fears. Was this, then, a manifestation of the workings of his unconscious? Was this an example of what Jung called the Shadow, that part of our personal or collective unconscious that we reject, suppress and deny? Did he, as he grew up through childhood, receive, as so many children do, daily bombardments of 'oughts' and 'shoulds' from the adults peopling his world and, with these, censure and disapproval if he fell short in any way. Were the authoritarian outside voices that said "bad boy" absorbed into his psyche so that he created an inner critic that simply carried on where the adults left off? Such voices could indeed sound demonic in situations of extreme stress such as those brought about by the prospect of dying. If you're somehow 'bad' then you deserve eternal punishment, say the relentless inner voices. Or then again, did he actually encounter evil in some form?

We think of diagnoses as clear, unalterable statements of fact. It is not so easy, as this story suggests. Three different lenses, three different explanations. Take your pick – or maybe combine them.

Gardens

Hospices give particular attention to nature. All the ones I have worked in have had gardens, which included water – in fountains, pools, streams or ponds – scented, flowering plants and bushes, shady places and bird feeders. Some palliative care units have raised flowerbeds so that patients in wheelchairs can do some gardening if they wish. Whenever I looked outside as I worked, I would see a few patients sitting in the sun and talking with their family. It was such an ordinary scene that I hardly took notice of it.

It was when I visited the Alhambra, the Moorish palace in Granada in Andalucia, Southern Spain, that I realised I had been missing something. No other palace I had seen had the same rich interweaving of nature and architecture. I moved from rooms to courtyards to gardens and back again, drinking in the extraordinary beauty of the place. The first rooms were decorated with wonderful tiles with endlessly repeating, multicoloured, geometric patterns. The plasterwork took up this theme with a kaleidoscope of shapes, seemingly abstract but hinting at natural themes such as stars, waves, trees and flowers. Interspersed with these forms were bas-relief extracts from the Qu'ran in flowing Arabic script. The proportions of each room were exquisite. Windows were not glazed so that cool air could flow freely into the rooms, but they continued the geometric theme in the form of plaster or wooden latticework.

Then there were the courtyards. There was the Court of the Lions with a circle of ancient, heraldic, stone lions guarding a central fountain which overflowed into four channels that streamed out like the points of the compass to cool the rooms which bordered the courtyard and were approached through a forest of slender, ornate columns. There was the Court of the Myrtles, enclosing a long, still, rectangular pool that mirrored the soft salmon-pink stone of the palace walls, the columns, the crenellated battlements and the myrtle bushes on either side. As I watched, a visitor put her hand into the water and ripples made the clear, geometric reflections wobble and distort pleasingly and then gradually die away to calmness again.

And the gardens: serried ranks of fountains rose and then fell into long, slender pools in which yellow-gold water lilies floated. A profusion of luxuriant, flowering bushes – glowing red, orange, yellow, mauve – grew alongside the water channels, accompanied by fruit trees, flowering plants and herbs. Tall cypress trees overshadowed the colonnaded walkways on either side. The scents of these plants – sweet, astringent, citrus, floral, pine – mixed with the smells of water on sun-heated earth and stone, while songbirds called in the foliage and pigeons flew down from time to time to drink from the pools.

The Moors were a desert people and they knew, better than any rain-swept Northern European could ever understand, just how precious water was, for with it came life, with it came herbs, foods and medicinal compounds. They tended their gardens with the utmost care. They created areas of cool shade as a protection from the heat of the sun. The Persians called them *pairidaeza*, paradise in English.

This same concern can be sensed in the description of the Garden of Eden by the authors of Genesis:

The Lord God planted a garden in Eden which is in the East... The Lord God caused to spring up from the soil every kind of tree, enticing to look at and good to eat, with the tree of life and the tree of the knowledge of good and evil in the middle of the garden. A river flowed from Eden to water the garden and from there it divided to make four streams.
(The Bible: Genesis. 2:8–10)

There are many other sacred gardens in myths and religious

traditions around the world: the Garden of the Hesperides, nymphs who tend a tree in the garden bearing golden apples of immortality; the Isle of Avalon where King Arthur is reputed to lie; the Elysian Fields in Greek mythology, the resting place of the souls of the virtuous; and the Pure Land, the celestial abode of a Bodhisattva or Buddha. Such gardens are secret and hard to find. They may be the place where lovers meet; they may be the dwelling place of the heart; they are an image of the soul; God himself is a garden. They represent the liminal space between the world of the spirit, the artifice of humanity and the wildness of nature.

These paradisiacal gardens are also places of safety. There is a painting by Edward Hicks, a 19th century American Quaker and folk artist called *The Peaceable Kingdom*. Actually, it was an obsession with him; he painted it 61 times in all, reflecting, perhaps, our deep human longing for a heaven-haven, as the poet, Gerard Manley Hopkins, called it. It shows young children, fearless among a throng of animals, including a lion, a tiger, a leopard, a bear and a wolf consorting peacefully with cattle, a goat and a lamb in a pastoral landscape. It refers to a prophecy from Isaiah:

> The wolf lives with the lamb,
> The panther lies down with the kid...
> With a little boy to lead them.
> (The Bible: Isaiah. 11: 6–9)

Yes, I had been missing something. When you sit in a garden, you are immersed in Life.

Murmurations

I was twelve and cycling along the towpath of the canal between the Exe estuary and Exeter. It was a late afternoon and the sky was an even, pale blue with the soft light that comes as the sun sinks to the western horizon. Then I heard a rustling in the distance. At first I took no notice but, as it grew louder, I stopped riding and turned to look around. Approaching me was the largest flock of starlings I had ever seen. They were so numerous that they were like a vast, dark cloud looming up from the south. Open-mouthed, I watched as this vast concourse flew past me. They were single-minded in their flight, heading north; I presumed they were flying to an inland roost. I don't know how long it took for the flock to pass for the simple reason that I had temporarily stepped outside the passing of time. My whole attention was in the now, observing this extraordinary spectacle. When they had gone, I, as it were, came down to Earth, and rode my bike slowly home, still taken up by what I had seen.

I later learned that when huge numbers of starlings fly down to roost in winter, this is called a murmuration. What a wonderful word. I saw this spectacle again a few years ago in Gloucestershire. As dusk fell, immense numbers of starlings flew in swirling clouds above the bare, black, silhouetted trees, forming and dissolving fluid patterns like the complex sound harmonics on an oscilloscope screen made in response to musical sounds fed into it. Enormous fan shapes would appear and disappear in moments and turn into swirling smoke blown in the wind. It was like the most complex dance routine, minutely choreographed; or it would recall natural shapes such as the ribbing of wet sand, or high sand dunes blown by the wind in the Sahara desert. Sometimes it was like dust clouds in arid country; or like ripples on water, waves at sea or whirlpools. Often it was similar to vast shoals of fish swirling and turning to avoid the predators which fed off them. Parts of the flock might break off, like dancers separating to perform their own solo, and then moments later become part of the main flock again. And yet none of these descriptions is adequate; none captures the lightning changes as the flock of maybe 80,000 birds circles in the air. And then, almost in a blink of an eye, they drop down to their perches in the trees, a gigantic, particulate, black funnel of starlings pouring out of the bleached, winter sky.

Starlings are thought to flock like this for survival: those on the periphery of the flock try to fly into the middle and so avoid being picked off by raptors such as peregrine falcons. How extraordinary, then, that something so instinctual should be endowed with so much beauty. It seems unnecessary for the task in hand; it achieves no evolutionary purpose. Maybe, then, there is a deeper imperative here than just survival.

In traditional accounts of Native Americans hunting, when they had killed their prey they prayed and asked the animal's forgiveness for taking its life, because they needed food to live. They respected their prey and believed that it let itself be taken in response to a divine imperative. The beauty of the animal, the thrill of the hunt, the rawness of death and the invocation to the Great Spirit all went hand in hand. No wonder their myths involve animals with supernatural powers – wily Coyote, shapeshifting Crow, gentle Deer, loyal Wolf, the sacred White Buffalo.

We are gifted with bifocal vision: at one level, we see the down-to-earth, stressful, gritty business of living and dying; at another level, we see with the eye of the soul. We may even – and this is hard – see through both lenses at once.

The starlings have something else to teach us. Their very lives depend on their intensely social nature. Listen to the clicking and twittering gossiping of roosting starlings. Watch how groups always forage together and respond together to alarm calls. They need each other.

And so, of course, do we. But you wouldn't believe it if you listen to talk of competition, individualism, winning or survival of the financial fittest. The truth is, as I once heard said, we need the cooperation of about a million other people just to get out of bed in the morning and go to work.

One of the strengths of hospices is that they are small. All in – patients, family, staff, home care – this will include maybe 50–150 people. This is about the size of traditional villages in many cultures, big enough to provide protection yet small enough to provide a close community. Our human social imperative is being met. Anyone walking into a hospice will tell you about its atmosphere – personal, cooperative and supportive. Imagine an old woman living alone in her tower block flat or an elderly man living by himself in a crime-ridden council estate. Admission to a palliative care unit must be a shock of relief. They are no longer isolated. They are among people again; people who relate to them.

Avian Synchronicities

One of the birds I most wanted to see when Joan and I visited the Pyrenees was the Lammergeier or Bearded Vulture. It is rare, difficult to find and only lives in remote mountainous areas. It is also huge, with a wingspan of nine feet, and it does indeed have a beard, two tufts of fine feathers that hang down either side of its beak. One of its trademark behaviours is to pick up a bone from a carcass it is eating, fly up in the air and drop the bone on to rock so that it smashes and the vulture can eat the fragmented pieces with their nutritious marrow. Its stomach acid is so powerful that it can even dissolve bone.

I didn't have any local knowledge so the most I could do was keep an eye out as we walked in the mountains. We saw dozens of Griffon Vultures, which are common in that area, but never a Lammergeier. It was very frustrating.

One day I decided to go exploring in the car. Following the advice of people who lived locally, I made my way slowly via steep hairpin bends up a narrow potholed road to the top of one of the mountain heights that surrounded the small village where we were staying. Then I drove back along a tiny, uneven road that hugged the side of the summit. On my left, there was a thousand foot drop to a valley far below, along which, like a silver thread, a river meandered. All the while I kept a lookout. Sometimes I stopped the car and scanned the vast panorama below me with my binoculars. Nothing. Looming dark grey clouds were gathering. It was going to rain – and hard. No self-respecting bird would want to be caught out in such a downpour. Feeling as gloomy as the clouds, I resigned myself to failure. As I drove, I saw a short track leading to a small clearing on my left. On a whim, I pulled the car in, got out my binoculars rather half-heartedly and walked to the edge of the clearing. As I surveyed the mountain falling steeply below me, I saw out of the corner of my eye on the left an enormous bird come sailing effortlessly round the shoulder of the mountainside. I knew it immediately – a Lammergeier, juvenile but still as big as an adult. I watched spellbound as it glided nonchalantly past me, not fifty feet away. I was so close I could see it turning its head from side to side, scanning the ground for dead animals. It kept close to the contours of the steep hillside it was patrolling and then, perhaps half a minute later, disappeared round a prominence to my right.

I stood there, not moving for some minutes, overcome by my good fortune. The timing was preternaturally perfect, the Lammergeier appearing just at the moment I arrived, almost as though it had been waiting for me. Had I turned up one minute later, I would have missed it. Ten minutes earlier and I wouldn't have waited. I would have been more than content with a snatched glance of a tiny Lammergeier speck floating high above me in the mountain air. Instead I had had a grandstand view at eye level. It was a marvellous gift.

I got back in the car. It started to rain. It became so heavy that I had to pull the car in because I couldn't see ahead. Happily I sat in the car listening to the drumming of the rain on the roof and looking at the blurred sheets of water pouring down the windscreen while I contemplated my good fortune.

There are many who would call this simply a coincidence, a chance coming together of circumstances. Not me. To me this was a gift. I have encountered too many wildly unlikely coincidences to believe there is no purposeful connection between them. Carl Jung described these as examples of synchronicity, which he defined as an acausal connecting principle. Further, the connection must be meaningful. He gave as an example the story of a middle-aged man who was seeing him for a neurosis. During one conversation, the man mentioned that, during the deaths of his wife's mother and grandmother, "a number of birds gathered outside the windows of the death-chamber." After the end of treatment, Jung sent this man to a heart specialist for suspected cardiac symptoms. Nothing was found. As the man walked home he collapsed in the street. He was taken home, dying. His wife was already very distressed because a flock of birds had alighted on their house soon after her husband went to the doctor. She wondered if someone was dying and her fears unhappily were soon confirmed. (Jung 1952, paras 843–5)

I'm reminded of how a guitar string will resonate with a musical note of the right pitch played by an instrument some distance from it. Perhaps, then, this is one way the Universe may work. When we hold a thought or intention, a kind of resonance may be created with the subject of our attention, facilitating the possibility, though not the certainty, of a coming together. If this seems unlikely we can turn for an analogy to the strange world of quantum theory. When two subatomic particles interact physically and then are separated by no matter how large a distance, they remain 'entangled' and continue to interact. When one begins to spin clockwise, the other, though it may be separated by billions of miles, will simultaneously start to spin either the same or the opposite way. True, thought intentions are not known to be the same as the forces of interaction between subatomic particles. However, there are other quantum experiments on subatomic particles which show that the simple fact of observation by the researcher will determine whether they behave as waves or particles: consciousness affecting physical reality. It gives an interesting new perspective on prayer which is predicated on just such an action.

The Chiffon Scarf

It is night. I am standing in the snow in Northern Canada looking up at the shimmering stars. The temperature is about -20°C. Across the sky far above the black tree-line sweep wave after wave of ever-changing curtains of light – soft green with tones of violet. It is like a vast chiffon scarf swirling in the wind, sometimes larger, sometimes fading away only to grow again. Its scale is huge and yet it is also evanescent. It is like a piece of visual music, one with no beginning and no end. I stand and watch, cold but entranced. Perhaps it is my imagination, but I think I hear a sound, a very faint, high-pitched hissing. Certainly it seems to fit with the spectacle. I feel very small, taken out of my little concerns at the sight of this extraordinary display, at once so delicate and yet so powerful. Eventually I am driven inside by the searching cold, but night after night I go out and watch the spectacle repeat itself, free for anyone to see. An overwhelming natural generosity.

There are myriad accounts of supernatural experiences, both within and without the major religious traditions around the world. Many of these are far outside our everyday human experience. Nevertheless, nature provides a wonderful resource whereby anyone may get in touch with a spiritual dimension within themselves. We need only attend. It doesn't take much. A flower, a leaf, a stone, a bowl of water; any of these will do. Go and look into a patient's room in a hospital or hospice and, almost without fail, there will be flowers there, or cards showing scenes from nature. If she is well enough to do some painting, she will most likely choose a pastoral scene or a still life of flowers. Or the patient may be outside in her wheelchair in a patch of garden enjoying the sun. Such simple things; but how rarely we give them our full attention, how rarely we truly value them.

Greeting the Divine

Joan and I woke very early, at 2.30 am. It was a 35 mile winding drive up the slopes of Mount Haleakala (the House of the Sun), the 10,000 foot dormant volcano that dominates Maui, one of the Hawaiian Islands, and we wanted to be in time to greet the sunrise from its heights at a little after 5 am. We wound up and up the hairpin bends, the lights of our car casting overlapping funnels of brightness into the dark; spreading trees, ferns and strange prehistoric palms loomed up, only to vanish as we passed them. The vegetation changed from tropical to something akin to Dartmoor. We drove on and up through the cloud layers, which fuzzed what little we could see. Showers of fine rain came and went continually, an effect of the prevailing winds blowing moist air off the sea and up the slopes of the volcano where it gave birth to the rainfall. The temperature at sea level was about 70° F; by the time we reached our destination, well above the cloud layer, it was not far from freezing. There was very little vegetation at this height; we were in a mineral world. A shooting star briefly blazed across the night sky seemingly threading its way between the stellar constellations. To our right, about a quarter of a mile away was a large observatory, its hemispherical nose gazing up into the depths of sidereal space. A chilly wind was blowing while we made our way in the darkness towards an eastern facing vantage point and joined others huddled in anoraks, blankets and duvets.

Slowly the night sky in the east paled. We began to see a soft, dove-grey blanket of clouds spreading out towards the eastern horizon with, here and there, a crag from the volcano's rim thrusting up above the cloud layer. Below us, the ground fell away steeply into the crater. Swirls of mist constantly moved with the prevailing wind revealing and then concealing the desolate interior of the volcano. Plant life seemed absent; instead there were mineral browns, greys, red earth, sands, indigo and muted greens. From time to time one of the many smaller eruption cones in the crater showed itself only to vanish again.

The horizon continued to brighten. Then the uppermost part of the rim of the sun rose above the clouds and the palest of brilliant, white-gold rays beamed out in a 180° arc. There was a collective sigh from those watching and cameras began to click, recording the sun's full circumference appearing in all its splendour.

Then, behind us and higher up on the rocks, I heard a man's voice singing, powerfully and skilfully. I recognised the pattern from other chants I had heard in Hawaii sung in their native language. It was a traditional invocation, greeting the rising of the sun god. It sounded a little like Native American chants and I found the hairs on the back of my neck standing up. I looked round. It was one of the park rangers, a Hawaiian, who was singing. He continued for a few minutes, ended, stood in silence for some seconds and then turned and walked away.

The sun, the source of our physical life, is represented in mythologies and religions around the world as a symbol of the divine, the source of our spiritual life. Thus in Greek mythology, Helios, the sun god, drives his flaming chariot across the heavens each day. Light, the emanation of the sun, becomes an emanation of the Spirit. We speak of holy men and women as being enlightened. A halo of light signifies such a person in many religions. When Christ was transfigured in the presence of his closest friends, "his face shone like the sun and his clothes became as white as light." (The Bible: Matthew. 17:2)

This is why the story of Esther does not surprise me. She was an elderly, white-haired Welsh woman who had widespread breast cancer and lymphoedema, or gross swelling, of her arm. She could scarcely lift it. She was deeply depressed about her condition and would be in tears, looking down at the floor and hardly able to speak for most of her meetings with the doctors. It was summertime and there was a spell of good weather. The nurses decided to wheel her, in her bed, down to the garden. There, accompanied by one of the nurses, she spent most of the day lying contemplating the white clouds sailing slowly by in the blue sky and the play of light and shadow on the grass and ornamental bushes nearby. She became pink from sunburn and a parasol was set up to protect her. She didn't want to do anything else. After two weeks, her depression had vanished.

Esther may not have thought consciously about the light in which she basked as an emblem of the sacred, but at a soul level perhaps she knew intuitively what she needed.

The Folly

From my home in Exeter, I could look out from my bedroom at a wonderful view that stretched as far as Haldon Hill, a high ridge between Exeter and Dartmoor. I could also see the cathedral to my right and, with the sun on its downward arc, the cathedral bells would peal their rounds while swifts chased each other, screaming in the clear air. Unless there was mist I could see a tower, tiny on the distant ridge of hills, silhouetted against the blue sky and surrounded by woods.

I remember visiting the tower as a child with my family. Then, it was very out of the way. You had to park your car in a narrow wooded lane and walk up a track overgrown with grass and weeds that sloped up diagonally from the road. There was some ineffective barbed wire (it only stretched halfway across the track) and an old sign with peeling paint informing would-be visitors of visiting hours and the charge (1s/3d or one shilling and thruppence). The tower was actually a Victorian folly. Two elderly reclusive brothers lived there. They were grey-haired, balding and wore old-fashioned clothes – collarless shirts, baggy corduroy trousers and sleeveless pullovers – while strong hob-nailed boots encased their feet. The whole of the ground floor of the folly was their living quarters. It was surprisingly spacious. There was a higgledy-piggledy clutter of old Victorian furniture and faded dusty oriental carpets, and display cabinets filled with stiff, stuffed animals set among twigs and moss in an attempt at realism. There was something rather ghostly about their fixed stares – especially the owl – which never changed from day to day. There was a quality of oldness, timelessness and silence in this circular living space. I had the feeling that the brothers didn't talk much – perhaps they knew each other so well they didn't need to. I think there were bedrooms leading off this main room. Having parted with our 1s/3d, we headed for a door to our left, opened it and found spiral stone stairs leading upwards. The walls were painted white and oblong slit windows punctuated our upward journey, letting in light to see by. It was a stiff climb, but well worth it. When we reached the top there was a flat roof surrounded by crenellated battlements. We looked over them and saw a vast vista of Devon. To the north and east lay Exeter spread out across the Exe valley while the river Exe itself meandered towards the sea, widening into a shining estuary. To the south and west we could see the hills of Dartmoor rising from its wooded flanks to emerge treeless and covered with gorses and heathers in purples, dark greens and yellows. Hay Tor, a grey volcanic outcrop of granite, stood as a silent witness to its ancient violent origins from subterranean, molten lava.

It felt easier to breathe up there. In the late afternoon there was a beautiful softness to the air and we could smell the damp woods below us and hear the wood pigeons repeatedly crooning their five note love song, or watch their courtship display: a steep ascent, wings flapping and clapping, and then a glide curving over an invisible, aerial hilltop and plunging down, wings held still and stiff, only to rise again in another parabola.

As soon as we can walk we start climbing; our first attempts on the household furniture graduate quickly to trees and climbing frames and then to hills, cliffs and mountains. Castles and towers are no different; they just have to be climbed. So do the Statue of Liberty and the Empire State Building in New York, and the Arc de Triomphe in Paris. As far as I know, mountain peaks don't hold any survival advantage so this urge to get to the top must originate elsewhere.

It is telling that in 1964 the psychologist Abraham Maslow used the term 'peak experiences' to describe states characterised by intense happiness, wonder, awe, harmony, ecstasy and inter-connectedness. Those overtaken by such elevated feelings may call them spiritual, mystical or religious. Somehow we associate heights with spiritual feelings, and this isn't new. Christians, Jews, Buddhists, Hindus and Native Americans, among others, have venerated particular mountains as holy for millennia.

Many years ago I came across a description by Carl Jung (1983 pp. 320–6) of his experiences following a heart attack when, as he put it, he "hung on the edge of death." He described an extraordinary vision in which he floated high in space. Below him was the Earth, "bathed in a gloriously blue light." He could see India, Ceylon (as it was then known), the Himalayas and the Arabian Peninsula. Then he saw an enormous block of stone the size of a house floating nearby. It was an Indian temple. As he approached it, he felt that "everything was being sloughed away... the whole phantasmagoria of human existence, fell away or was stripped from me – an extremely painful process." In the temple he was told he had to return to Earth and at that moment the vision ceased. He found the greatest difficulty in returning to the restrictive "box system" of everyday life again. Everything he saw about him was as nothing compared with his ineffable vision. Life seemed to him like a prison. During the weeks of recovery that followed, his days unfolded in "a strange rhythm." By day he felt weak and depressed, by night he experienced again the sense of floating in space, a bliss too wonderful to be described. He felt an inexpressible sanctity in the room.

It is no surprise, then, that we climb mountains. Up there, a little closer to the stars, even if we don't articulate it to ourselves, we just might find our heart's desire.

The Music of the Thing That Is

One Good Friday Joan, my son and I go to a performance of Bach's St John Passion at the Barbican in central London. Our seats are near the back and I look down the stepped rows of seats – all filled – and listen to the orchestra tuning up and watch the players adjusting their instruments until discord becomes accord. Then, to applause, the conductor and soloists appear.

There is that moment of silent, pregnant expectation when the conductor has raised his baton, and the soloists sit quietly, the men in white tie and the women in formal evening gowns, and the orchestra is poised, bows on strings, lips to woodwinds. Then, as his baton arcs in the air, the music appears seemingly out of nowhere and we are transported by the familiar dissonant solemn first chords into a sacred story of a man's passion – which means suffering in the original sense of the word – and death. Even though it is a concert hall performance, it has the feel of a religious ritual being enacted.

The singing is perfect. Each note is clear, each voice in harmony. I feel I can trust the sounds I hear, I can let them in, they are true to what the composer intended. I and the music, in all its extraordinary beauty, gradually become as one. The singing is like waves flowing across the sea and lapping on a beach, or like the sound of the wind in the trees. For long periods I experience timelessness. Then something catches my eye or ear, a movement in the audience or a cough, and, for a little, I am back in chronological time again, only to float back once more into the eternal present.

At the end there is silence, as if the audience is still under the spell of the music. Then applause echoes around the hall; a clapping thank you where the sharp percussions fizz like hail on a tin roof. I feel still and calm. The music has elevated a story of violent judicial murder to something more: a tale of tragedy, love, grief, grandeur and redemption.

As I think back on that night, I wonder about the other people in the audience. There were, I would guess, about 1000 people there. There were probably a good number of card-carrying Christians, but there would also have been a wide mixture of other persuasions – atheists, agnostics and members of non-Christian religions. If I could have brought them together again to discuss their views on the story of Christ's crucifixion, there would very shortly have been a Babel of voices and contradictory opinions. But, at the level of our experience of the performance, there would, I think, have been far greater unanimity. We might all have used words like beautiful, moving, uplifting, inspiring; we might all have agreed it is a work of genius; we might even have used words like spiritual or soulful, even if one person would have understood these in a secular way and another in a sacred manner. In this divided world, I take comfort from that possibility. Experience is true – and can be shared even when beliefs differ.

The ill and dying people I have talked to over the years have voiced an astonishing variety of views on spiritual matters, reflecting the world at large. At the level of experience, however, it is different. They may talk of the blessed relief of being free of pain, or of being able to breathe more easily, or of being able to sleep better. They may mention their anxiety about being a burden for their partner. They may recall with sadness the death of a close friend. They may feel anger at falling ill. They may wonder what it is like to die. They may speak of their joy at being reunited with an estranged member of their family. They may rediscover simple pleasures: sitting in the garden on a sunlit day; a piece of music; a hot bath; looking at family photographs.

Every one of these is a human experience with which, as fellow human beings, we can empathise. We, too, have had like experiences. To me, they are also profoundly spiritual, but maybe what is important is, not the words, but the shared reality. I came across a passage once from Irish mythology in which the poet and warrior Oisin is asked what music he likes best. He replies that it is the music of the thing that is.

The Sound of Silence

As I walked into Westminster Cathedral that evening, I saw that it was full, but not in the ordinary sense of the word implying that all the chairs were taken. It was more than that – there was a person sitting on every square foot of the floor. The cathedral was carpeted with human beings. I had never seen anything like it; there must have been 5000 people there. At the same time the sound of singing softly embraced me. It sounded somewhat like Benedictine, or perhaps Russian Orthodox, chanting. The sound had a sonorous depth and power to it that only a huge number of voices singing in unison could provide. I could feel it rising up into the gloom of the shadowy heights above us and then reflecting down again. The cathedral was in darkness apart from candles. Hundreds of them had been placed on every available flat surface such as the altar railings, the pulpit and candle-holders lit before statues. They cast a mellow glow quite unlike the glare of electrical light.

I found the effect awe-inspiring and quite beautiful. In a happy daze, I wandered down the left-hand aisle, picking my way between the sitting singers towards the front. I could see that in front of the sanctuary there was a large Byzantine crucifix, perhaps six feet long, resting on the ground and surrounded by candles. I found a space and sat down. As I listened, I realised that the same phrase was being repeated over and over again, sometimes louder, sometimes softer. There was a small orchestra playing in accompaniment. Soon I was able to discern what was being sung and could join in. It was very simple. I could feel myself entering the timelessness of this meditative chanting. After quarter of an hour or so a new chant started, this time in Latin. Later, another was sung as a round. If the singing had been powerful so far, the effect of introducing harmonies was yet more evocative. It reminded me of shoals of glinting fish swimming in ever-changing patterns. So in the cathedral the different groups of voices sent their harmonies up into the space above us, where they swirled around each other and descended again to our receptive ears.

I can't remember how long the service went on but I travelled home in what could fairly be described as an altered state of consciousness, my being still in synchrony with the sacred sounds we had all created.

This event had been conceived by a group from Taizé, an ecumenical religious community in South-Western France, where such singing plays a major part in their services.

In my mind's eye I recall entering a patient's room. He is asleep. The French windows look out on to a sunny courtyard with raised flowerbeds and trailing vines. A radio by his bed is quietly playing Classic FM – I presume this must be his favourite channel.

This is a scene that I have encountered many times. The music might differ – perhaps jazz, Big Band, forties music or even Taizé chants – but the intent is the same: music to bring calmness, relaxation, healing, pleasure. A refuge during a difficult time. Perhaps no one notices. don't we all have the radio on much of the day? But when you are very ill or dying, the extraneous tends to drop away. It's the so-called little things that become important. And for some people this is music.

A Birthright

We were standing on a huge spur of rock jutting out into the Grand Canyon. The still, evening air had a soft, clear radiance and we could smell the subtle scents of the still-warm rocks, earth, trees and flowers. Occasionally a raven flew past far below us, its deep croaking reaching us a fraction after it had called. To our left, the sun was sinking towards the western horizon. To our right, since the canyon is orientated in an east-west direction, the continually changing angle of the sunlight cast ever-varying patterns of blue-grey shadows on the salmon coloured rocks of this vast rift. There were about a hundred people watching and there were convenient iron railings near the edge to stop anyone falling the mile or so to the bottom of the canyon.

After a while, I noticed something unusual. Normally a crowd is noisy with chatter, people moving around, a sort of restless energy. But here it was not like that. Instead, people for the most part sat quietly watching the natural display before them and if they talked it was *sotto voce*, like birds settling to roost at night. They were absorbed by the beautiful spectacle before them and it seemed their rhythms synchronised with the slow, subtle onset of dusk. It reminded me of something and for a while I couldn't think what it was. Then I had it. Spontaneously, unpremeditated, we had moved into sacred consciousness. It was like the experience of sitting in Chartres Cathedral or listening to Mozart's *Magic Flute* or becoming absorbed in the colours of a Cézanne painting. Here, unbidden, was the experience people miss when they make their spirituality an onerous duty. By contrast this felt light, free and spacious. This crowd was no different to any other, and yet these people were able to slip into an altered state with no effort. Such happenings, then, are not the preserve of the few. They are, in fact, everyone's birthright.

In one hospice I worked in, a bird feeder was placed just

outside the windows of one of the wards. Some of the patients would sit for hours and watch the activities of the blue tits, great tits and chaffinches flitting on and off the feeder. Very simple and easy to miss. Nothing spectacular. Yet contemplative in its own way. And pleasurable as well. Enlightenment is happy to use the most ordinary of everyday events. All we need to do is turn up, be aware and look; so often we don't.

The Miz-Maze

Overlooking Winchester is a hill, St Catherine's Hill, crowned by an Iron Age fort. Joan and I and our three children, along with Ben, our enthusiastic golden retriever, used to go there sometimes. It was a steep climb up the fields to the top of the hill where we could see a large grove of trees surrounded by a defensive wall and ditch. Over the centuries these had been softened by the elements: the wall had been worn down to an easily climbed hump and the ditch had been gradually filled in by erosion and an annual influx of dead leaves. We would climb over and walk through the quiet, wooded, inner sanctum of the fort, while Ben would run ahead full of excitement, alternately sniffing and peeing a calling card for the next dog. There had once been a medieval chapel dedicated to St Catherine in the centre of the stronghold. It now lay under a cluster of trees known locally as the Clump.

Just beyond the fort on a flat piece of meadow, there is a maze called the Miz-Maze. It is big, about 90 feet in diameter and, unlike most mazes which are circular, is square with rounded edges. It was constructed by cutting the turf away to reveal the earth pathways. It is thought to be about 300 years old. On one occasion, as we walked towards the maze, I noticed beautiful sprays of spring flowers placed among the branches of some saplings nearby. It was just after the spring equinox. The old religion, I thought; still quietly kept alive by its devotees. I felt touched to see this simple gesture of fidelity and yet uneasy as though there were some ancient, invisible presence watching.

The maze itself was our chief purpose and we would, one by one, set off on our labyrinthine journeys winding in towards the centre and out again to the periphery. The odd thing was that you might meet someone ahead of you whose path had curved back to meet yours only to find that suddenly you had diverged again and were at opposite ends of the maze. With a group of people walking the Miz-Maze there was a repeating process of meeting and parting, only to meet again. It is an apt metaphor for life – the same meeting and parting and meeting again. Journeying around the maze had a strange rather surreal feel to it as if we were travelling on two planes, one material and the other archetypal. Journey's end, the place we did all meet eventually was the Centre, the Heart of the labyrinth.

This Centre is not just a concept. It describes a personal reality. We all have an individual Centre, or perhaps it is closer to the truth to say that this Centre has us. We might call it our Heart, our Soul, the Self, the Still Point, the Place of Silence, the Knower or the Void. We are all on a journey to this place, even if we don't know we are. When life seems to be utterly dark, it may be that we are very close, just one step away from our Truth; just as in the labyrinth, when we have yet again circled far out to the periphery, we may suddenly come upon the final part of the path that leads us straight to the Centre.

That phrase "Heart to Heart" really is true. When you speak from your Heart, your Centre, then you speak to the Heart, the Centre, of others. St Teresa of Avila used a beautiful metaphor to describe the soul – she called it an Interior Castle, shining, crystalline and transparent. In concentric circles there are a series of dwelling places, one inside the other. Our life journey is to reach the inmost – here is the wellspring of love. Often, it is a hard, long, perilous way to find this place. But it is worth it. It is what we were born for. And it is what we die for.

Conclusion

Everyone experiences some degree of illness and suffering. Everyone wants to heal. It is not enough, however, to think of ourselves as machines which can be serviced like a car and which can be put right with a spare part. While this has been a wonderfully useful paradigm, it has its limits.

When one part of us is ill, all the other parts are affected. Body, mind, feelings, soul and relationships all interact, or perhaps we should say "inter-are" to borrow a word from the Vietnamese Buddhist monk, Thich Nhat Hanh. So often, attempts at healing fail because this truth is not remembered. The words 'healing' and 'whole' have the same root and this isn't by chance.

When death comes – and it will come to all of us – it doesn't have to be an enemy to be fought off at all costs. It might even be a friend. We can heal in life and we can heal in death.

The legend of the phoenix is found in many cultures. It is a bird of extraordinary beauty and gorgeous song. Every thousand years the phoenix, sometimes called the firebird, builds a nest and sets itself ablaze. Both bird and nest are reduced to ashes, leaving an egg from which a new phoenix arises. I think this is a beautiful way of saying that nothing is lost. Dying holds within it the necessity of rebirth. Whether we think our life continues in heaven or through our children or through the legacy we leave behind or is recycled into other forms of life, we continue, part of an immense, glittering, timeless web of light.

Notes

Introduction

1. Kava is a euphoriant drink made from the dried roots of the tropical kava plant.

Chapter 1

2. There are a number of theories explaining spontaneous remission of cancer. Some patients' cancers disappear after an infection, suggesting stimulation of the immune system by the infection; others improve after changes in their thyroid, oestrogen and growth hormone levels; some improve after developing high temperatures; others' tumours regressed after they outgrew their blood supply; some reports indicate tumour regression through mind-body interaction such as visualisation; finally, there are many carefully documented reports of inexplicable healings from cancer considered to be miraculous.

Chapter 6

3. Cardinal Hume was Archbishop of Westminster; he died in 1999.

Chapter 9

4. In French, *Satan* is pronounced with equal stress on both syllables. Both a's are spoken as in 'hallo'.

References

Arnott, A. (1983) *Secret Country of CS Lewis*. Basingstoke: Lakeland

Attar, FU-D (1984) *The Conference of the Birds*. Trans. A. Darbandi and D. Davis. London: Penguin

Axline, V. (1971) *Dibs: In Search of Self*. Harmondsworth: Pelican

Barwick, D. (1998) *Rebellion at Coranderrk*. Canberra: Aboriginal History Inc.

Blake, W. (1970) *Songs of Innocence and Experience*. Oxford: Oxford University Press

Blake, W. (1994) *The Selected Poems of William Blake*. London: Wordsworth Editions Ltd.

The Bible (1966) *The Jerusalem Bible*. London: Darton, Longman and Todd

Bloom, Metropolitan A. (1971) *God and Man*. London: Darton, Longman and Todd

Brewster, D. (1855) *Memoirs of the Life, Writings, and Discoveries of Sir Isaac Newton (Volume II)*. Edinburgh: Constable

Buber, M. (1961) *Between Man and Man*. London: Fontana

Byrne, L. (2008) *Angels in my Hair*. London: Century

Campbell, J. (1990) *The Hero's Journey*. Novato, CA: New World Library

Chambers (1988) *Chambers Dictionary of Etymology*. Edinburgh: Chambers

Chödrön, P. (1997) *When Things Fall Apart*. London: Element

Clottes, J. (ed.) (2003) *Return to Chauvet Cave*. London: Thames & Hudson

Dickinson, E. (1924) *The Complete Poems of Emily Dickinson*. London: Martin Secker

Donne, J. (1839) *The Works of John Donne. Vol. III*. H. Alford, ed. London: John W. Parker

Ellis, B. (1981) *The Long Road Back*. Great Wakering: Mayhew-

McCrimmon

Frankl, V. (2004) *Man's Search for Meaning*. London: Rider

Giono, J. (1954) *The Man Who Planted Trees*. London, Peter Owen

Homer (1919) *The Odyssey. Vol. 1*. Trans. AT Murray. London: William Heinemann

Itard, JMG (1802) *An Historical Account of the Discovery and Education of a Savage Man, or of the First Developments, Physical and Moral, of the Young Savage Caught in the Woods Near Aveyron in the Year 1798*. London: Richard Phillips

Jerome, St (1933) *Select Letters*. Trans. FA Wright. London: Harvard University Press

Johnson, R. (1998) *Balancing Heaven and Earth*. New York: HarperSanFrancisco

Jung, C. (1952) "Synchronicity: An Acausal Connecting Principle". In: H. Read, M. Fordham and G. Adler, eds. (1953–1979) *The Collected Works of CG Jung. Vol. VIII*. London: Routledge

Jung, C. (ed.) (1964) *Man and his Symbols*. London: Aldus

Jung, C. (1983) *Memories, Dreams, Reflections*. London: Flamingo

Jung, C. (1984) *Modern Man in Search of a Soul*. London: Ark

Lawrence, Brother (2006) *The Practice of the Presence of God and the Spiritual Maxims*. New York: Cosimo

Lewis, CS (1963) *The Magician's Nephew*. Harmondsworth: Penguin

Katie, B. and Mitchell, S. (2002) *Loving What Is*. London: Rider

Katie, B. and Katz, M. (2005) *I Need Your Love – Is That True?* London: Rider.

Mandela, N. (1995) *Long Walk to Freedom*. London: Abacus

Melville, J. and Schwarz, C. (1990) *St Christopher's Hospice*. London: Together Publishing Company and St Christopher's Hospice.

Milgram, S. (1974) *Obedience to Authority: An Experimental View*. London: HarperCollins

Moody, RA (1976) *Life After Life*. New York: Bantam

Neihardt, JG (1988) *Black Elk Speaks.* Lincoln and London: University of Nebraska Press

Noonan, P. (2006) "The Sounds That Still Echo From 9/11". *The Wall Street Journal.* September 9, 2006. http://online.wsj.com /article/SB11577470 4992357920.html (accessed 18.08.13)

Porter, R. (1997) *The Greatest Benefit to Mankind: A Medical History of Humanity From Antiquity to the Present.* London: Fontana Press

Proust, M. (2006) *Remembrance of Things Past: Vol. II.* Trans. CK Scott Moncrieff and S. Hudson. Ware, Herts: Wordsworth Editions

Rinpoche, S. (1992) *The Tibetan Book of Living and Dying.* London: Rider

Santayana, G. (1905) *The Life of Reason. Vol. 1: Reason in Common Sense.* New York: Scribner

Schweitzer, A. (1948) *On the Edge of the Primeval Forest & More from the Primeval Forest.* London: Adam & Charles Black

Scott, GF (ed.) (2002) *Selected Letters of John Keats: Revised Edition.* Cambridge, Mass: Harvard University Press

Shakespeare, W. (1905) *Hamlet.* In: WJ Craig, ed. *Shakespeare Complete Works.* London: Oxford University Press

Sherrington, CS (1942) *Man On His Nature.* Cambridge: Cambridge University Press

Simonton, O., Matthews-Simonton, S. and Creighton JL (1986) *Getting Well Again.* London: Bantam

Solnit, R. (2013) *The Faraway Nearby.* London: Granta

Sydenham, T. (1848) *The Works of Thomas Sydenham, M.D. Translated from the Latin Edition of Dr. Greenhill, with a Life of the Author by R.G. Latham M.D. Vol I.* London: The Sydenham Society

Ten Boom, C. (2005) *Tramp for the Lord.* London: Hodder & Stoughton

Tolle, E. (1999) *The Power of Now.* London: Hodder and Stoughton

Williams, M. (2004) *The Velveteen Rabbit.* London: Egmont

Williams, WC (1967) *The Autobiography of William Carlos Williams*.
New York: New Directions

Yancey, P. and Brand, P. (1997) *The Gift of Pain*. Grand Rapids,
Michigan: Zondervan

AYNI
BOOKS

"Ayni" is a Quechua word meaning "reciprocity" – sharing, giving and receiving – whatever you give out comes back to you. To be in Ayni is to be in balance, harmony and right relationship with oneself and nature, of which we are all an intrinsic part. Complementary and Alternative approaches to health and well-being essentially follow a holistic model, within which one is given support and encouragement to move towards a state of balance, true health and wholeness, ultimately leading to the awareness of one's unique place in the Universal jigsaw of life – Ayni, in fact.